Handbook of Treatment-resistant Schizophrenia

Handbook of Treatment-resistant Schizophrenia

Leslie Citrome
New York Medical College
Valhalla, NY

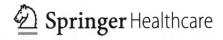

Published by Springer Healthcare Ltd, 236 Gray's Inn Road, London, WC1X 8HB, UK.

www.springerhealthcare.com

© 2013 Springer Healthcare, a part of Springer Science+Business Media.

British Library Cataloguing-in-Publication Data.

A catalogue record for this book is available from the British Library.

ISBN 978-1-908517-86-9

Project editor: Tess Salazar
Designer: Joe Harvey
Artworker: Sissan Mollerfors
Production: Marina Maher
Printed in Great Britain by Latimer Trend

Contents

Author biography

Leslie Citrome, MD, MPH, is Clinical Professor of Psychiatry & Behavioral Sciences at New York Medical College, Valhalla, NY, and was the founding Director of the Clinical Research and Evaluation Facility at the Nathan S. Kline Institute for Psychiatric Research in Orangeburg, NY. After nearly two decades of government service as a researcher on the psychopharmacological treatment of severe mental disorders, Dr Citrome is now engaged as a consultant in clinical trial design and is a frequent lecturer on the quantitative assessment of clinical trial results using the evidence-based medicine metrics of number needed to treat and number needed to harm. Dr Citrome graduated from the McGill University Faculty of Medicine in Montreal, Quebec, Canada, and completed a Residency and Chief Residency in Psychiatry at the New York University School of Medicine. He went on to complete a Masters in Public Health from the Columbia University School of Public Health in New York City. Dr Citrome's primary research interests have centered on psychopharmacologic approaches to schizophrenia, management of treatment-refractory schizophrenia, and the management of aggressive and violent behavior. He is the author or coauthor of over 400 research reports, reviews, chapters, and abstracts in the scientific literature. He is the Deputy Editor and incoming Editor-in-Chief for the *International Journal of Clinical Practice*, serves on the editorial board of six other medical journals, reviews for over 50 journals, and has lectured extensively throughout the United States, Canada, Europe, and Asia.

Disclosures

No writing assistance was used in the production of this handbook. In the past 36 months, Leslie Citrome has engaged in collaborative research with or received consulting or speaking fees from: Alexza, Alkermes, AstraZeneca, Avanir, Bristol-Myers Squibb, Eli Lilly, Envivo, Forest, Genentech, Janssen, Lundbeck, Merck, Mylan, Novartis, Noven, Otsuka, Pfizer, Shire, Sunovion, and Valeant.

Abbreviations

BPRS	Brief Psychiatric Rating Scale
CATIE	Clinical Antipsychotic Trials of Intervention Effectiveness
CBT	cognitive-behavioral therapy
CDSS	Calgary Depression Scale for Schizophrenia
CGI-I	Clinical Global Impressions–Improvement scale
CGI-S	Clinical Global Impressions–Severity scale
EBM	evidence-based medicine
ECT	electroconvulsive therapy
FDA	US Food and Drug Administration
HAM-D	Hamilton Depression Rating Scale
HDRS	
HRSD	
MADRS	Montgomery-Åsberg Depression Rating Scale
MCCB	MATRICS Consensus Cognitive Battery
NMDA	*N*-methyl-d-aspartate
NNH	number needed to harm
NNT	number needed to treat
NSA-16	Negative Symptom Assesment-16
PANSS	Positive and Negative Syndrome Scale
PSP	Personal and Social Performance scale
rTMS	repetitive transcranial magnetic stimulation
SANS	Scale for the Assessment of Negative Symptoms
SAPS	Scale for the Assessment of Positive Symptoms
UPSA	UCSD Performance-based Skills Assessment
YMRS	Young Mania Rating Scale

Preface

The aim of this handbook is to provide an overview of the management of schizophrenia, focusing on the patient with an apparent suboptimal treatment response. This may include outpatients who are dissatisfied with the progress they are making, patients who seem to have frequent relapses, or hospitalized patients receiving intermediate- and long-term care. There is a high degree of heterogeneity among patients with schizophrenia in terms of clinical course, intensity of symptoms, degree of functional impairment, comorbid conditions, and response to medication. The adage "one size fits all" does not apply to schizophrenia.

This book should appeal to clinicians who are involved in the day-to-day treatment of patients with schizophrenia and who desire a systematic framework in which they can plan their interventions. The book is divided into two parts. Part One provides an overview of the factors that a clinician ought to consider before categorizing a person with schizophrenia as "treatment-resistant." The first chapter provides an overview of schizophrenia that includes definitions of response, remission, and recovery, and the measurement tools commonly used in clinical trials and reported in journal articles. The second chapter follows with a primer on the philosophy and practice of evidence-based medicine, the importance of the therapeutic alliance, the potential use of motivational interviewing, and a strategy for identifying barriers to care. Adherence, alcohol and substance use, and optimal dosing are then discussed in the context of being the most common roadblocks to treatment response.

Part Two provides information on treatments that can be considered for patients with schizophrenia who are treatment-resistant despite monotherapy with antipsychotics at appropriate doses for an adequate period of time, and where adherence is not in question. Data on psychopharmacological, psychological, and behavioral strategies are discussed in terms of both promise and limitations, with emphasis on results from controlled clinical trials and meta-analyses. This includes exciting new work regarding glutamatergic pathways in the brain that impact on dopamine neurotransmission.

This book is the result of a 25-year career, almost all of it spent in public mental health systems in the United States on the federal, state, and county levels as a clinician, researcher, and educator. Instilling hope and avoiding therapeutic nihilism is the responsibility of everyone who is involved in the care of patients with schizophrenia.

PART ONE

Before categorizing someone as treatment-resistant

Chapter 1

Introduction

Overview

Schizophrenia is a common chronic mental disorder estimated to have a global prevalence of about 0.5–1.0% in the general population and a prevalence of 1.0% in the US population [1,2]. Typically, people with schizophrenia initially present for treatment when they have their first acute psychotic episode. This usually occurs in a patient's teens or early adulthood. Response to antipsychotic medication during the first episode is usually robust in terms of reduction of positive psychotic symptoms, such as hallucinations and delusions, and the hope is to forestall further deterioration in overall functioning. The duration of untreated psychosis prior to the initiation of treatment has been linked to poor prognosis with poorer symptomatic and functional recovery in initial episodes [3]. In addition, subsequent psychotic episodes are generally more difficult to treat, requiring longer periods of time before symptoms diminish [4]. Negative symptoms and cognitive impairments are less likely to substantially improve. Interruption of antipsychotic medication treatment is common and adds to the difficulties in managing this illness. Stigma, poverty, homelessness, and poor access to care all add to the observation of "downward drift" as the disease becomes chronic and symptoms endure.

Because resolution of symptoms is usually incomplete, one can make the case that all persons with schizophrenia are potentially treatment-resistant. Over time, treatment response is even more difficult

L. Citrome, *Handbook of Treatment-resistant Schizophrenia*,
DOI: 10.1007/978-1-908517-88-3_1,
© Springer Healthcare 2013

to achieve [4]. Selection of therapies for people with schizophrenia who are partially responsive or refractory to treatment can be complex. The research that supports evidence-based clinical decision-making has used a variety of definitions of treatment-resistance as it relates to psychopathology, severity of symptoms, symptom dimensions, functionality, remission, and recovery. Clinical obstacles to optimal care include adherence, comorbid disorders such as substance use, and the selection of an appropriate dose of antipsychotic medication. This handbook aims to classify the principal issues in the identification and management of persons with treatment-resistant schizophrenia, including the role of first-generation antipsychotics, second-generation antipsychotics (with an emphasis on clozapine), antipsychotic combination therapies, augmentation of antipsychotics with other types of medications, and nonpharmacological interventions, including somatic treatments (eg, electroconvulsive therapy) and psychological options (eg, cognitive remediation).

Definitions

Treatment-resistance or treatment-refractoriness is in the eye of the beholder. A person with treatment-resistant schizophrenia may be distressed because of residual anxiety and poor sleep, but the clinician may be more concerned with a patient's persistent florid delusions and hallucinations. Parents may be more worried about their son or daughter staying in their room all day, for example, smoking cigarettes and having no motivation to do anything else. All of these aspects of the illness deserve attention, but not all are equally amenable to treatment.

Ultimately, a compromise will need to be made, as no single intervention is perfect. In order for a medication to be effective in the "real world," it must be efficacious enough to target the most important symptoms (from all perspectives), be tolerated "well enough" in that the patient does not object to the adverse events that invariably arise, be considered "safe enough" so that the clinician is comfortable in prescribing it, and the patient has to be sufficiently adherent. Adherence is never perfect; an operational research definition of adequate adherence is typically the taking of at least 80% of the prescribed dose [5].

In this context, research definitions of treatment-refractory schizophrenia have been formulated. These definitions attempt to operationalize treatment-resistant schizophrenia so that potential interventions can be tested in a clinical trial. For example, in the pivotal clinical trial used to support regulatory approval of clozapine for treatment-resistant schizophrenia, potential subjects not only had to meet DSM-III criteria for schizophrenia, but also the following requirements [6]:

- A history of at least three periods of treatment in the preceding 5 years with antipsychotic medication agents from at least two different chemical classes at doses equivalent to or greater than 1000 mg/day of chlorpromazine for a period of 6 weeks (each without significant symptomatic relief).
- No period of good functioning within the preceding 5 years.
- A certain threshold of psychopathology as determined by the Brief Psychiatric Rating Scale (BPRS) and the Clinical Global Impressions–Severity (CGI-S) scale. Item scores of at least moderate were required on two of the following four BPRS items: conceptual disorganization, suspiciousness, hallucinatory behavior, and unusual thought content.

Moreover, patients who met both the historical criteria for treatment-resistance and the initial severity criteria were also required to fail a 6-week prospective period of treatment with haloperidol to confirm the lack of drug responsiveness [6]. Improvement in this context was defined as a 20% decrease in the BPRS total score plus either a post-treatment CGI-S rating of mildly ill or a post-treatment BPRS score of 35 or less. The assumption was made that the prior trials of antipsychotics were legitimate with adequate adherence, and that failure as such was not attributable to poor tolerability but to inadequate symptom relief [6]. The prospective trial of haloperidol used a dose of approximately 60 mg/day, considerably higher than what would be considered optimal today, to ensure that only patients who were truly treatment-resistant could enter the trial. All of these requirements for eligibility for randomization to receive clozapine are clearly in excess to what takes place today in current clinical decision-making when evaluating patients for clozapine therapy.

Subsequent clinical trials in treatment-resistant schizophrenia have used more relaxed entry criteria. For example, an outpatient study that examined the efficacy of clozapine included people with a DSM-III-R diagnosis of schizophrenia or schizoaffective disorder and living in the community or judged clinically treatable in the community despite psychotic symptoms [7]. Partial or poor response was defined by documented treatment failure in two trials of conventional antipsychotics at doses equivalent to or greater than chlorpromazine 600 mg/day for at least 6 weeks and one trial of a conventional agent at doses equivalent to chlorpromazine 250–500 mg/day for the same length of time. Patients for whom a low-dose trial could not be documented received prospective dose reduction for 4 weeks, or less if clinical worsening was seen. Patients were required to rate at least moderate on one of the following four BPRS items: conceptual disorganization, suspiciousness, hallucinatory behavior, and unusual thought content.

The term "suboptimal treatment response" rather than "treatment-resistance" was employed in a study that compared clozapine, olanzapine, risperidone, and haloperidol [8]. For inclusion in the study, patients were required to have a diagnosis of DSM-IV chronic schizophrenia or schizoaffective disorder and suboptimal response to previous treatment, which was defined by two criteria that needed to be present:

1. Persistent positive symptoms (hallucinations, delusions, or marked thought disorder) after at least 6 contiguous weeks of treatment, presently or documented in the past, with one or more typical antipsychotics at doses of at least 600 mg/day in chlorpromazine equivalents.

2. Poor level of functioning over the past 2 years, defined by the lack of competitive employment or enrollment in an academic or vocational program and not having age-expected interpersonal relations with someone outside the biological family of origin with whom ongoing regular contacts were maintained.

In addition, patients were required to have a baseline total score ≥60 on the Positive and Negative Syndrome Scale (PANSS). Patients were excluded from the study if they had a history of nonresponse to clozapine, risperidone, or olanzapine, defined as an unambiguous lack of improvement despite a contiguous adequate trial of risperidone or olanzapine for at least 6 weeks or clozapine for at least 14 weeks. No prospective period of treatment to confirm lack of drug responsiveness was required [8].

The Clinical Antipsychotic Trials of Intervention Effectiveness (CATIE) for schizophrenia used a pragmatic approach for initial study entry and a broad effectiveness measure as the primary study outcome. Outpatients with schizophrenia were eligible for Phase I with only a few exclusions [9]. If patients discontinued Phase I because of inadequate efficacy, they were encouraged to enroll in the Phase II part of the trial, which included potential randomization to open-label clozapine or double-blinded olanzapine, risperidone, or quetiapine [10]. Treatment-resistance was not formally assessed other than by virtue of having failed Phase I because of efficacy concerns as judged by the investigator. Realistically, this is probably the closest to what occurs in day-to-day clinical practice.

Thus, over time, research studies that have examined the use of antipsychotic medications for treatment-resistant schizophrenia have differed and evolved in their operational definitions of treatment-resistance. In addition, the field has begun to recognize and appreciate the complex multidimensional aspects of schizophrenia and its treatment. In particular, much work is underway regarding the measurement and treatment of negative symptoms and cognitive dysfunction, aspects of schizophrenia that are probably more disabling than the presence of hallucinations and delusions [11]. Moreover, the symptom domains of depression and anxiety may be of particular interest and concern to the individual patient, impacting both the therapeutic alliance (between the clinician and the patient) and medication adherence if left ignored; the symptom domain of excitement/hostility has been a frequent reason for hospitalization. In essence, lack of treatment-response or treatment-resistance can be either global or restricted to a specific domain.

Measurement tools

Several research instruments are in common use when comparing the efficacy of different antipsychotics and other medications for the treatment of schizophrenia. The BPRS, CGI-S, and PANSS have been mentioned earlier as they have been used in studies of treatment-resistant schizophrenia. Table 1.1 outlines these and other psychopathology rating scales commonly used in clinical trials of patients with schizophrenia [12]. The PANSS has been extensively analyzed using 5-factor models that have identified independent treatment domains: positive, negative, excitement, cognitive, and depression/anxiety factors [13,14]. As noted, for many patients, targeting positive symptoms is a high priority, but for still many others it may be negative and cognitive symptoms or excitement and hostility. Different antipsychotics may be advantageous depending on the specific target symptoms [15] with perhaps the best example being clozapine's superior efficacy in managing hostility, aggression, and violent behavior [16].

The PANSS has largely supplanted the use of the BPRS in clinical research trials of schizophrenia. Nonetheless, the PANSS is not amenable

Scale	Abbreviation	Number of items	General use
Brief Psychiatric Rating Scale	BPRS	18	Psychopathology in psychotic disorders
Calgary Depression Scale for Schizophrenia	CDSS	9	Depressive symptoms
Hamilton Depression Rating Scale	HAM-D or HDRS or HRSD	17	Depressive symptoms (not used as often as the CDSS or MADRS in studies of schizophrenia)
Montgomery-Åsberg Depression Rating Scale	MADRS	10	Depressive symptoms; also often used in studies of major depressive disorder and bipolar disorder
Negative Symptom Assesment-16	NSA-16	16	Negative symptoms in schizophrenia; this is a shortened version of the original scale
Positive and Negative Syndrome Scale	PANSS	30	Psychopathology in psychotic disorders
Scale for the Assessment of Negative Symptoms	SANS	20	Negative symptoms in schizophrenia
Scale for the Assessment of Positive Symptoms	SAPS	30	Positive and disorganized symptoms in schizophrenia
Young Mania Rating Scale	YMRS	11	Manic symptoms

Table 1.1 Psychopathology rating scales, an abbreviated list. Adapted from Rush et al [12].

to regular use in a clinic setting for the routine management of patients. It requires some degree of training in order to use it [17,18], even with the availability of a structured interview and rating manual. Completion of the PANSS can take an average of 45 minutes for the interview and additional time to score its 30 items. A high score can be driven by positive symptoms, negative symptoms, or general psychopathology, and hence these subscales need to be looked at separately along with the total PANSS score.

In contrast to the PANSS, the CGI-S and its counterpart, the CGI-Improvement (CGI-I) scale, are simple, intuitive, quick, and clinically relevant [19]. Table 1.2 outlines the scoring for each of these two measures [19]. With some caveats, the CGI-S has been shown to correlate reasonably well with the PANSS [20,21]. It would be useful for the clinician to use this scale as a means of tracking progress, or lack thereof. The CGI construct has been adapted to focus on a variety of specific outcomes, such as positive, negative, depressive, and cognitive symptoms [22] as well as efficacy, safety and tolerability, and an "integrated" outcome that explicitly includes both efficacy and safety/tolerability [23].

Cognition in clinical trials of schizophrenia can be formally assessed using neuropsychological testing. The standard today is to use a battery of tests called the MATRICS Consensus Cognitive Battery (MCCB). The MCCB consists of ten tests designed to evaluate performance across seven

Clinical Global Impressions–Severity and –Improvement	
Clinical Global Impressions–Severity (CGI-S)	**Clinical Global Impressions–Improvement (CGI-I)**
Considering your total clinical experience with this particular population, how mentally ill is the patient at this time?	Compared to his/her condition at admission to the project, how much has he/she changed?
0 = Not assessed	0 = Not assessed
1 = Normal, not at all ill	1 = Very much improved
2 = Borderline mentally ill	2 = Much improved
3 = Mildly ill	3 = Minimally improved
4 = Moderately ill	4 = No change
5 = Markedly ill	5 = Minimally worse
6 = Severely ill	6 = Much worse
7 = Among the most extremely ill patients	7 = Very much worse

Table 1.2 Clinical Global Impressions–Severity and –Improvement. Adapted from Guy [19].

domains: speed of processing, attention/vigilance, working memory, verbal learning, visual learning, reasoning and problem solving, and social cognition [24]. At present there are no clinician-friendly bedside tests that can be easily and quickly administered to assess cognition other than gross measures of cognitive ability such as the Mini-mental State Examination [25].

Functional impairment is probably more clinically relevant than focusing exclusively on psychopathology or on the results of cognitive testing alone. In this context, any residual symptoms that cause distress or impairment in personal, social, or occupational functioning, despite several treatment attempts, can be interpreted as evidence for treatment-resistance. Although functional impairment can be driven by symptoms, it has been observed that 5–17% of patients who experience functional recovery do not demonstrate symptomatic remission [26].

There are several research tools available to assess and quantify psychosocial functioning. These scales include the Personal and Social Performance (PSP) scale [27,28] and the UCSD Performance-based Skills Assessment (UPSA) [29]. The PSP has been used as a prespecified secondary outcome measure for agents undergoing regulatory approval, hence PSP outcomes can appear in product labeling [30]. The PSP includes four domains: socially useful activities, including work and study; personal and social relationships; self-care; and disturbing and aggressive behaviors. The latter domain, and the PSP total score, may be heavily influenced by the presence of positive symptoms including hostility. The UPSA is performance-based with five domains of functioning: household chores, communication, finance, transportation, and planning recreational activities. Administration of the UPSA requires about 30 minutes. UPSA performance correlates with severity of negative symptoms and cognitive impairment but not with positive or depressive symptoms. Agents undergoing regulatory approval in the United States for the indication of cognitive improvement in schizophrenia require that both cognitive testing and an assessment of functioning be used as co-primary outcomes [31]. In contrast, agents undergoing regulatory approval for the indication of negative symptoms in schizophrenia do not require a co-primary outcome of functionality.

Remission

In contrast to major depressive disorder and bipolar mania, where definitions of remission have been tethered to maximum thresholds in single rating scale scores, working definitions of remission in schizophrenia are more complex [32]. Symptomatic remission can be defined as the maintenance over a 6-month period of simultaneous ratings of mild or less on delusions, hallucinations, disorganized speech, grossly disorganized or catatonic behavior, and negative symptoms, as defined by the PANSS, BPRS, Scale for Assessment of Positive Symptoms (SAPS), or Scale for Assessment of Negative Symptoms (SANS). There are no items in these scales related to patient goals, desires, preferences, or values; cognitive and functional outcomes were not included in this first iteration from the Remission in Schizophrenia Working group that authored this proposal [32].

Symptomatic remission may be difficult to achieve and maintain. In the CATIE trial, at baseline 16.2% of patients were in symptomatic remission [33]. Across the medication phases of the trial, only 11.7% attained and then maintained at least 6 months of symptomatic remission, and 55.5% (n = 623) did not experience symptom remission at any visit.

A model for functional remission has been proposed [34]. Domains include productive activities, residential and self-maintenance activities, and social relationships. Criteria include level of accomplishment (from none to full success) and breadth of accomplishment across functional domains (from making progress in one domain to full success in three domains) [34].

Recovery

Recovery is a process, not an endpoint. Social outcomes play a key role [35–38]. Adequate symptom remission, vocational functioning, independent living, peer relationships, and duration of at least 2 years are some of the proposed components of recovery [36,37]. A cure or absence of illness is not realistic, but being in recovery is. The proponents of the recovery movement emphasize the process of managing illness more effectively, having a meaningful life in the community, and moving ahead with one's life despite illness [38]. Table 1.3 outlines the highlights of two well-articulated models of recovery [35,39,40]. In terms of hierarchies of desired endpoints, recovery is at the top and assumes some degree of remission and stability.

Summary

Schizophrenia is a chronic mental illness that ordinarily becomes more difficult to treat over time. Resolution of symptoms is usually incomplete and there is significant disability. Lack of treatment-response or treatment-resistance can be either global or restricted to a specific domain. Measurement tools include psychopathology rating scales, neuropsychological testing, and assessments of functional impairment. Perhaps the most clinician-friendly measurement tools are the CGI-S and CGI-I. Goals of treatment are for a clinically relevant decrease in symptoms (response), minimization of symptoms (remission), and being in recovery.

Highlights of two models of recovery

Davidson's Nine Common Elements of Recovery	Substance Abuse and Mental Health Services Administration's Ten Fundamental Components of Recovery
1. Renewing hope and commitment	1. Consumer self-direction
2. Redefining self	2. Individualized and person-centered treatment
3. Incorporating illness into life as a whole	3. Empowerment
4. Involvement in meaningful activities	4. An holistic treatment focus
5. Overcoming stigma	5. A nonlinear perspective of change
6. Assuming control	6. Treatment focused on strengths instead of deficits
7. Becoming empowered and exercising citizenship	7. The inclusion of peer support in treatment
8. Managing symptoms	8. Respect for consumers and consumer self-respect
9. Finding social support	9. Consumer acceptance of personal responsibility
	10. Hope in recovery

Table 1.3 Highlights of two models of recovery. Adapted from Peebles et al [35], Davidson et al [39], US Department of Health and Human Services Substance Abuse and Mental Health Services Administration Center for Mental Health Services [40]. Copyright © 2005 by the American Psychological Association. Adapted with permission. The official citation that should be used in referencing this material is Davidson L, O'Connell MJ, Tondora J, Lawless M, Evans AC. Recovery in serious mental illness: a new wine or just a new bottle? Prof Psychol Res Pr. 2005;36:480-487. The use of APA information does not imply endorsement by APA.

References

1   Andreasen NC, Black DW. *Introductory Textbook of Psychiatry.* 4th ed. Washington, DC: American Psychiatric Publishing, Inc., 2006.

2   American Psychiatric Association. *Diagnostic and Statistical Manual of Mental Disorders DSM-IV-TR Fourth Edition (Text Revision).* Arlington, VA: American Psychiatric Association; 2000.

3   Perkins DO, Gu H, Boteva K, Lieberman JA. Relationship between duration of untreated psychosis and outcome in first-episode schizophrenia: a critical review and meta-analysis. *Am J Psychiatry.* 2005;162:1785-1804.

4   Lieberman JA, Alvir JM, Koreen A, et al. Psychobiologic correlates of treatment response in schizophrenia. *Neuropsychopharmacology.* 1996;14(3 suppl):13S-21S.

5   Velligan DI, Weiden PJ, Sajatovic M, et al. The expert consensus guideline series: adherence problems in patients with serious and persistent mental illness. *J Clin Psychiatry.* 2009;70(suppl 4):1-46.

6   Kane J, Honigfeld G, Singer J, Meltzer H. Clozapine for the treatment-resistant schizophrenic. A double-blind comparison with chlorpromazine. *Arch Gen Psychiatry.* 1988;45:789-796.

7   Kane JM, Marder SR, Schooler NR, et al. Clozapine and haloperidol in moderately refractory schizophrenia: a 6-month randomized and double-blind comparison. *Arch Gen Psychiatry.* 2001;58:965-972.

8   Volavka J, Czobor P, Sheitman B, et al. Clozapine, olanzapine, risperidone, and haloperidol in the treatment of patients with chronic schizophrenia and schizoaffective disorder. *Am J Psychiatry.* 2002;159:255-262.

9   Lieberman JA, Stroup TS, McEvoy JP, et al; Clinical Antipsychotic Trials of Intervention Effectiveness (CATIE) Investigators. Effectiveness of antipsychotic drugs in patients with chronic schizophrenia. *N Engl J Med.* 2005;353:1209-1223.

10 McEvoy JP, Lieberman JA, Stroup TS, et al; CATIE Investigators. Effectiveness of clozapine versus olanzapine, quetiapine, and risperidone in patients with chronic schizophrenia who did not respond to prior atypical antipsychotic treatment. *Am J Psychiatry.* 2006;163:600-610.

11 Kurtz MM. Symptoms versus neurocognitive skills as correlates of everyday functioning in severe mental illness. *Expert Rev Neurother.* 2006;6:47-56.

12 Rush AJ Jr., First MB, Blacker D, eds. *Handbook of Psychiatric Measures.* 2nd ed. Arlington, VA: American Psychiatric Publishing, Inc; 2008.

13 Lindenmayer JP, Czobor P, Volavka J, et al. Effects of atypical antipsychotics on the syndromal profile in treatment-resistant schizophrenia. *J Clin Psychiatry.* 2004;65:551-556.

14 Lehoux C, Gobeil MH, Lefebvre AA, Maziade M, Roy MA. The five-factor structure of the PANSS: a critical review of its consistency across studies. *Clin Schizophr Relat Psychoses.* 2009;3:103-110.

15 Citrome L, Bilder RM, Volavka J. Managing treatment-resistant schizophrenia: evidence from randomized clinical trials. *J Psychiatr Pract.* 2002;8:205-215.

16 Volavka J, Citrome L. Heterogeneity of violence in schizophrenia and implications for long-term treatment. *Int J Clin Pract.* 2008;62:1237-1245.

17 Opler LA, Ramirez PM. Use of the positive and negative syndrome scale (PANSS) in clinical practice. *J Practical Psychiatry Behavior Health.* 1998;4:157-62.

18 Opler LA, Opler MG, Malaspina D. Reducing guesswork in schizophrenia treatment. *Curr Psychiatry.* 2006;5:76-78, 81-82, 84.

19 Guy W. *ECDEU Assessment Manual for Psychopharmacology Revised, 1976.* Rockville, MD: US Department of Health, Education, and Welfare, National Institute of Mental Health; 1976. DHEW publication (ADM) 76-338.

20 Levine SZ, Rabinowitz J, Engel R, Etschel E, Leucht S. Extrapolation between measures of symptom severity and change: an examination of the PANSS and CGI. *Schizophr Res.* 2008;98:318-322.

21 Leucht S, Kane JM, Etschel E, Kissling W, Hamann J, Engel RR. Linking the PANSS, BPRS, and CGI: clinical implications. *Neuropsychopharmacology.* 2006;31:2318-2325.

22 Haro JM, Kamath SA, Ochoa S, et al; SOHO Study Group. The Clinical Global Impression-Schizophrenia scale: a simple instrument to measure the diversity of symptoms present in schizophrenia. *Acta Psychiatr Scand Suppl.* 2003;(416):16-23.

23 Targum SD, Pestreich L, Reksoprodjo P, Pereira H, Guindon C, Hochfeld M. A global measure to assess switching antipsychotic medications in the treatment of schizophrenia. *Hum Psychopharmacol.* 2012;27:455-463.

24 Nuechterlein KH, Green MF, Kern RS, et al. The MATRICS Consensus Cognitive Battery, part 1: test selection, reliability, and validity. *Am J Psychiatry.* 2008;165:203-213.

25 Folstein MF, Folstein SE, McHugh PR. "Mini-mental state". A practical method for grading the cognitive state of patients for the clinician. *J Psychiatr Res.* 1975;12:189-198.

26 Figueira ML, Brissos S. Measuring psychosocial outcomes in schizophrenia patients. *Curr Opin Psychiatry.* 2011;24:91-99.

27 Morosini PL, Magliano L, Brambilla L, Ugolini S, Pioli R. Development, reliability and acceptability of a new version of the DSM-IV Social and Occupational Functioning Assessment Scale (SOFAS) to assess routine social functioning. *Acta Psychiatr Scand.* 2000;101:323-329.

28 Nafees B, van Hanswijck de Jonge P, Stull D, et al. Reliability and validity of the Personal and Social Performance scale in patients with schizophrenia. *Schizophr Res.* 2012;140:71-76.

29 Patterson TL, Goldman S, McKibbin CL, Hughs T, Jeste DV. UCSD Performance-Based Skills Assessment: development of a new measure of everyday functioning for severely mentally ill adults. *Schizophr Bull.* 2001;27:235-245.

30 Invega® (paliperidone) [package insert]. Titusville, NJ: Janssen Pharmaceuticals, Inc.; 2011.

31 Harvey PD, Bowie CR. Cognitive enhancement in schizophrenia: pharmacological and cognitive remediation approaches. *Psychiatr Clin North Am.* 2012;35:683-698.

32 Andreasen NC, Carpenter WT Jr, Kane JM, Lasser RA, Marder SR, Weinberger DR. Remission in schizophrenia: proposed criteria and rationale for consensus. *Am J Psychiatry.* 2005;162:441-449.

33 Levine SZ, Rabinowitz J, Ascher-Svanum H, Faries DE, Lawson AH. Extent of attaining and maintaining symptom remission by antipsychotic medication in the treatment of chronic schizophrenia: evidence from the CATIE study. *Schizophr Res.* 2011;133:42-46.

34 Harvey PD, Bellack AS. Toward a terminology for functional recovery in schizophrenia: is functional remission a viable concept? *Schizophr Bull.* 2009;35:300-306.

35 Peebles SA, Mabe PA, Davidson L, Fricks L, Buckley PF, Fenley G. Recovery and systems transformation for schizophrenia. *Psychiatr Clin North Am.* 2007;30:567-583.

36 Liberman RP, Kopelowicz A. Recovery from schizophrenia: a concept in search of research. *Psychiatr Serv.* 2005;56:735-742.

37 Liberman RP, Kopelowicz A, Ventura J, Gutkind D. Operational criteria and factors related to recovery from schizophrenia. *Int Rev Psychiatry.* 2002;14:256-272.

38 Davidson L, Schmutte T, Dinzeo T, Andres-Hyman R. Remission and recovery in schizophrenia: practitioner and patient perspectives. *Schizophr Bull.* 2008;34:5-8.

39 Davidson L, O'Connell MJ, Tondora J, Lawless M, Evans AC. Recovery in serious mental illness: a new wine or just a new bottle? *Prof Psychol Res Pr.* 2005;36:480-487.

40 US Department of Health and Human Services Substance Abuse and Mental Health Services Administration Center for Mental Health Services. National consensus statement on mental health recovery. www.store.samhsa.gov/shin/content//SMA05-4129/SMA05-4129.pdf. Published 2006. Accessed March 19, 2013.

Chapter 2

A general treatment approach

Using the rubric of evidence-based medicine

Evidence-based medicine (EBM) is not just about the evidence, but how to use it in a meaningful way [1]; practicing EBM is not "cookbook medicine." Sackett et al [2] have summarized this well: "EBM is the conscientious, explicit and judicious use of current best evidence in making decisions about the care of individual patients." As such, there is a need to integrate individual clinical experience and expertise with external evidence. This evidence can be from a variety of sources and not necessarily from meta-analyses or randomized controlled trials. Key to this process is incorporating the individual patients' values and preferences.

External evidence that focuses on "effectiveness" may be the most useful, and "pragmatic clinical trials" may more closely resemble clinical practice. Effectiveness can be defined as how well an intervention will work in the "real world." In order to be effective, an intervention needs to be efficacious (ie, reduce symptoms), tolerable and safe (ie, not be associated with problematic side effects), and the patient has to be adherent [3]. Outcome measures such as time to all-cause discontinuation can serve as a proxy measure for effectiveness because continuation of a medicine is dependent on efficacy, tolerability, and adherence [4]. In contrast, randomized controlled trials used for regulatory approval of new medications often have strict inclusion and exclusion criteria that can render generalizability of the results difficult. Moreover, the principal outcome measure is ordinarily focused on a narrow definition of efficacy such as

L. Citrome, *Handbook of Treatment-resistant Schizophrenia*,
DOI: 10.1007/978-1-908517-88-3_2,
© Springer Healthcare 2013

reduction from baseline on a rating scale score such as the Positive and Negative Syndrome Scale (PANSS). In these trials, tolerability and safety is tested among relatively healthy individuals with a minimum of comorbid conditions, which is quite a different situation from what practitioners can typically expect to encounter in the clinic. Nonetheless, in the absence of relevant pragmatic effectiveness trials, the availability of other evidence can still be informative, provided that the trial limitations are acknowledged.

EBM makes clinical decision-making explicit; Figure 2.1 illustrates the 5 steps in the EBM process [5]. Formulating the question accurately will aid in productive online searches for possible answers. Appraising the evidence will require the clinician to ensure that the research is relevant to the patient at hand. Familiarity with concepts such as number needed to treat and number needed to harm will aid in the determination of clinical relevance of results that are statistically significant [6]. Applying the results and assessing the outcome are the final steps and need to be patient-centered.

The therapeutic alliance

Without a therapeutic alliance, adherence is challenging, communication between clinician and patient is subpar, and outcomes are poor. A therapeutic alliance involves three essential components: tasks (in-therapy behaviors and cognitions that form the therapeutic process); goals (mutually endorsed and valued, and are the targets of an intervention); and bonds (the patient–therapist attachment that includes mutual trust, acceptance, and confidence) [7]. This collaborative bond between therapist and patient can enhance treatment effectiveness through safe and supportive interaction, psychoeducation, and the involvement of the patient in the prescribing process rather than the patient simply receiving the prescription. In patients with schizophrenia it may be difficult to determine if rapport has been established as negative symptoms may mask it. Also, cognition may make understanding of basic disease concepts difficult; lack of insight generally interferes with a patient's ability to recognize many potentially disabling symptoms. The challenge is thus to identify what is important and understandable to the patient and to build from there. This can include feelings of anxiety and anger that the patient

The 5-step evidence-based medicine process

Step 1   Formulate the question

What kind of patient or problem?

What intervention, treatment, diagnostic test, risk factor, or prognostic factor are you interested in?

What comparisons are you making (treatment A versus treatment B, treatment versus no treatment, etc.)?

Step 2   Search for answers

Does it work?

Has a systematic review been conducted (search Medline or the Cochrane Database)?

Are there RCTs that enrolled similar patients to yours?

If using guidelines, are they evidence-based or eminence-based?

Well formulated questions make it easier to locate an answer, if one exists.

Step 3   Appraise the evidence

Will it work in the "real world"?

Is it relevant to your question and your patient?

Is the statistically significant result clinically significant?

If effect size is not mentioned in the research report, is there sufficient information available to calculate the NNT for the categorical outcomes of interest?

Step 4   Apply the results

Is it worth it?

Is the intervention, treatment, diagnostic test, etc., important to you within the context of your clinical experience and important to the patient in terms of their preferences?

Step 5   Assess the outcome

Did you ask the right question?

Did you find answers?

Were the answers you found based on a high-quality level of evidence?

Did it make clinical sense?

Did it make a difference?

Can you quantify this?

Does the patient agree?

Figure 2.1 The 5-step evidence-based medicine process. NNT, number needed to treat; RCT, randomized clinical trial. Reproduced with permission from Citrome and Ketter [5].

can more easily articulate, or a patient's wants or desires that appear to be thwarted. This can include issues regarding being able to sleep late in the morning, favorite foods, desire to have more funds, or a place to live. Asking innocuous questions about sleep and appetite can be a good tactic before discussing more emotionally laden topics. It is particularly important to avoid appearing judgmental regarding unpleasant personal habits, minor legal infractions, or other behaviors, otherwise a clinician may be less likely to hear about potentially clinically relevant information.

A therapeutic alliance is essential in order to be able to practice EBM. One of the key components of EBM is integrating a patient's values and preferences into medical decision-making.

Motivational interviewing

Motivational interviewing is a treatment technique that builds upon a therapeutic alliance and further develops it as a means to elicit change. Motivational interviewing is a patient-centered and directive therapeutic style that increases the potential to resolve ambivalence and change behaviors. A central concept is exploring the patient's own motivations for change [8]. A meta-analysis of motivational interviewing outcomes in 72 clinical trials spanning a range of target problems found effect sizes that were highly clinically relevant in the short-term and somewhat less robust in the long-term [9].

Motivational interviewing has been used to develop insight or coping skills, and helps make changes in health-related behaviors in patients with schizophrenia [10], including adherence [11] as well as comorbid substance use disorders [12]. Motivational interviewing has been proposed as a foundation for "recovery-oriented care" [13].*

Identifying obstacles

Obstacles to treatment response, remission, and recovery can fall under several categories [14] and should be reviewed as an essential part in the general treatment approach:

---

*A full discussion of motivational interviewing is beyond the scope of this handbook and the reader is urged to consult the Motivational Interviewing website at www.motivationalinterview.org for additional resources.

- Patient-related issues, including:
  - poor insight;
  - a negative attitude toward interventions, including medication;
  - cognitive impairment;
  - negative symptoms;
  - poor language skills; and
  - active alcohol or substance use.
- Treatment-related issues, including:
  - side effects of medications; or
  - inadequate reduction of symptoms.
- Environmental and relationship-related issues, including:
  - absence of a supportive family environment;
  - lack of social supports in the community;
  - problems with the therapeutic alliance with any of the clinicians involved in the care of the patient; and
  - practical problems in getting to appointments; paying for medication; or other barriers to access to care.
- Societal-related barriers, including the stigma attached to:
  - having a mental disorder; and
  - visibly obvious medication side effects such as abnormal motor movements, sedation, or substantial weight gain.
- Clinician barriers, including:
  - underestimating the importance of the therapeutic alliance;
  - the conveyance of hopelessness; and
  - the lack of interest in the life goals and other issues important to the patient.

Having a mental checklist is useful in order to systematically assess these obstacles for each individual patient. All of these barriers can impact the patient's adherence [15] and ultimately their response, remission, and recovery.

Summary

The philosophy of EBM takes into account a clinician's experience and the patient's values and preferences. It also makes explicit the process of searching for, appraising, and implementing evidence-based treatment recommendations. The therapeutic alliance is central to this process of medical decision-making. Motivational interviewing builds upon a therapeutic alliance and further develops it as a means to elicit change. The identification of treatment obstacles and the skillful resolution of them are important in the assessment and treatment of people with schizophrenia.

References

1   Citrome L. Evidence-based medicine: it's not just about the evidence. *Int J Clin Pract.* 2011;65:634-635.
2   Sackett DL, Rosenberg WM, Gray JA, Haynes RB, Richardson WS. Evidence-based medicine: what it is and what it isn't. *BMJ.* 1996;312:71-72.
3   Citrome L. Efficacy versus effectiveness. In Kattan MW, ed. *Encyclopedia of Medical Decision Making.* Thousand Oaks, CA: Sage Publications, Inc.; 2009:431-433.
4   Lieberman JA, Stroup TS, McEvoy JP, et al; Clinical Antipsychotic Trials of Intervention Effectiveness (CATIE) Investigators. Effectiveness of antipsychotic drugs in patients with chronic schizophrenia. *N Engl J Med.* 2005;353:1209-1223.
5   Citrome L, Ketter TA. Teaching the philosophy and tools of evidence-based medicine: misunderstandings and solutions. *Int J Clin Pract.* 2009;63:353-359.
6   Citrome L. Compelling or irrelevant? Using number needed to treat can help decide. *Acta Psychiatr Scand.* 2008;117:412-419.
7   Bordin E. Theory and research on the therapeutic working alliance: new directions. In: Horvath A, Greenberg L, eds. *The Working Alliance: Theory, Research, and Practice.* New York, NY: John Wiley & Sons; 1994:13-37.
8   Miller WR, Rollnick S. *Motivational Interviewing: Helping People Change.* 3rd ed. New York, NY: The Guilford Press; 2013.
9   Hettema J, Steele J, Miller WR. Motivational interviewing. *Annu Rev Clin Psychol.* 2005;1:91-111.
10 Baier M. Insight in schizophrenia: a review. *Curr Psychiatry Rep.* 2010;12:356-361.
11 Barkhof E, Meijer CJ, de Sonneville LM, Linszen DH, de Haan L. Interventions to improve adherence to antipsychotic medication in patients with schizophrenia–a review of the past decade. *Eur Psychiatry.* 2012;27:9-18.
12 Lubman DI, King JA, Castle DJ. Treating comorbid substance use disorders in schizophrenia. *Int Rev Psychiatry.* 2010;22:191-201.
13 Flaum M. Motivational interviewing as a foundation for "recovery-oriented care". *Community Psychiatrist.* 2011;25:8.
14 Pitschel-Walz G, Bäuml J, Bender W, Engel RR, Wagner M, Kissling W. Psychoeducation and compliance in the treatment of schizophrenia: results of the Munich Psychosis Information Project Study. *J Clin Psychiatry.* 2006;67:443-452.
15 Velligan DI, Weiden PJ, Sajatovic M, et al. The expert consensus guideline series: adherence problems in patients with serious and persistent mental illness. *J Clin Psychiatry.* 2009;70(suppl 4):1-46.

Chapter 3

Adherence – the great masquerader of treatment-resistance

What is adherence and how common is partial or nonadherence?

Adherence or compliance with a medication regimen is generally defined as the extent to which patients take medications as prescribed [1]. The term "compliance" has fallen out of favor as it implies a power imbalance between clinician and patient. The pejorative labeling of a patient as "noncompliant" is not therapeutically productive. The term "adherence" is more consistent with a shared decision-making model and the establishment of a therapeutic alliance. It is common in research studies of adherence to categorize a patient as adherent if they take at least 80% of their prescribed medication [2].

Because nonadherence can be viewed as failure, there is a consistent bias to overestimate adherence and underestimate nonadherence [3]. In the case of schizophrenia, clinicians may assume lack of adequate response to medication as "treatment-resistance" and thus lack of efficacy for the antipsychotic for that patient. This is a possible explanation for the common use of high dosing of antipsychotics, polypharmacy with other antipsychotics, and combination treatment with anticonvulsants [3,4]. This of course is a no-win cycle: adherence is even more of a challenge with complex regimens.

Nonadherence and partial adherence to antipsychotic medication treatment is common and has been observed in about half or more of all patients with schizophrenia [5–8]. It is estimated that about 75% of patients with schizophrenia become nonadherent within 2 years of

L. Citrome, *Handbook of Treatment-resistant Schizophrenia*,
DOI: 10.1007/978-1-908517-88-3_3,
© Springer Healthcare 2013

hospital discharge [9]. Adherence behavior can change and fluctuate over time and should be considered part of the illness [10].

Clinical correlates for people at risk for partial or nonadherence

As discussed in the prior chapter, adherence can be impacted on by patient-, clinician-, medication-, environmental/relationship-, and societal-related factors. Patient-related risk factors for nonadherence include poor insight, prior nonadherence, negative views of medication treatments, active substance use problems, and cognitive impairment. Cognitive impairment can result in communication difficulties and misunderstanding of instructions for medication administration, and may also be associated with difficulties in learning from experience. A robust therapeutic alliance can address some of the issues related to negative attitudes toward treatment. The strength of a therapeutic alliance correlates with medication adherence, as evidenced in a landmark study of 143 patients with schizophrenia showing that patients who formed good alliances with their therapists within the first 6 months of treatment were significantly more likely to remain in psychotherapy, comply with their prescribed medication regimens, and achieve better outcomes after 2 years, with less medication, than patients who did not [11].

Lack of insight is frequently encountered among patients with schizophrenia, with one review stating that between 50% and 80% of the patients diagnosed with schizophrenia were shown to be partially or totally lacking insight into the presence of their mental disorder [12]. Although patients with schizophrenia can have limited insight into their psychotic symptoms, patients can retain insight in other ancillary symptoms, such as impaired sleep, anxiety, and dysphoria. Thus, from a patient's point of view, a medication that has reduced the intensity and frequency of auditory hallucinations and delusions but has not alleviated poor sleep, anxiety, or dysphoria will be considered by the patient as unhelpful to them; this can also lead to nonadherence, eventual worsening of the psychotic symptoms, and the mistaken belief on the part of the clinician that the patient is refractory to treatment [13].

Treatment-related issues include adverse events of medications or inadequate reduction of symptoms. Key factors are the level of distress experienced by the patient rather than the actual severity, and the attribution of the adverse event and subsequent distress to the medication. This experiential component can vary from patient to patient even though the objective examination (such as the observation of tremor) is the same. Thus, one patient may become nonadherent because of a specific adverse event whereas another patient might not. The most commonly associated adverse events observed with partial or nonadherence are weight gain, sedation, akathisia, sexual dysfunction, parkinsonian symptoms, and cognitive problems [2].

With regard to treatment-related side effects, clinicians and patients may have very different attitudes and opinions regarding their importance [14]. The main factor influencing patient response to a side effect is their subjective distress. The more the patient is distressed, the less likely adherence will occur. This distress may appear out of proportion to the side effect (mild tremor, sedation, or weight gain). Ultimately, when considering adherence attitudes, patient belief is always reality [10]. Clinicians may be more impressed by the objective severity of the side effect and the potential impact on safety and risk. An example is potentially clinically relevant elevations in lipids and/or glucose for which the patient may show little concern or interest. Side-effect profiles do need to be considered when selecting treatment and need to balance an individual patient's preferences together with minimizing risks for long-term excess morbidity and premature mortality [2,15].

Partial or nonadherence may also be attributable to environmental- and relationship-related issues such as the absence of a supportive family environment or, at the very least, someone available to help monitor and assist with adherence. In addition, there may be people in the patient's family and social environment who lack a basic understanding of mental disorders and thus minimize the importance of medication therapy when interacting with the patient. There may be practical issues such as the lack of transportation to appointments, to the pharmacy, or a place to safely store the medications where they can be easily retrieved. There may be delays in filling prescriptions because of prior authorization requirements or there may be, unbeknownst to the prescriber, a substantial copayment.

Alcohol and substance use

Alcohol and substance use can confound the assessment of treatment-resistance both directly (exacerbation of positive or negative symptoms) and indirectly (through partial or nonadherence). In a prospective study of risk factors for nonadherence to antipsychotics in the treatment of schizophrenia, the top three predictors of nonadherence, ordered by strength of association, included prior nonadherence, recent illicit drug use, and recent alcohol use [16].

An estimated one-half of all individuals with schizophrenia use alcohol or illicit substances [17]. Several hypotheses have been suggested to explain this [18], including the possibility that:
- schizophrenia leads to substance use;
- substance use leads to schizophrenia;
- substance use and schizophrenia have a common origin;
- the increased rate of substance use results from multiple risk factors, including affect dysregulation and poor coping skills; and
- substance use is a response to reward circuitry dysfunction.

Lifetime prevalence of any alcohol use disorder diagnosis was estimated to be 34% among people with schizophrenia included in the Epidemiologic Catchment Area study of the National Institute of Mental Health [17]. Prevalence of any other drug use disorder diagnosis was estimated to be 28% [17]. Among patients enrolled in the Clinical Antipsychotic Trials of Intervention Effectiveness (CATIE) trial [19], laboratory testing elicited positive results for all tested drugs in 28% of subjects, with cocaine use in 16%, marijuana use in 15%, opiate use in 3%, and stimulant use in 2% of participants [20]. In the CATIE trial, about 11% of subjects were categorized as having moderate/severe substance use; significantly poorer outcomes were observed in the domains of psychosis, symptoms of depression, and quality of life for moderate/severe drug users in comparison with both mild users and abstainers [21].

Interview style

One of the basic tools available to clinicians treating people with mental disorders is the interview process, which can promote and encourage adherence. The interview style becomes critically important in this context. The first step is to destigmatize missing and/or stopping medication use. It is useful to acknowledge that virtually everyone misses or stops using medications, not just the mentally ill. Rather than ask, "Have you been taking your medications?" or "You have been taking your medicines, right?" it is more fruitful to start with, "Everyone misses doses of their medicines. Can you give me some idea of how many doses you usually miss in any given week? I just need a ballpark figure. You don't have to be exact." This is followed by, "What doses do you miss the most: mornings? Evenings? With meals? In between meals? This way we can figure out the best time of day to use these medications so we can minimize the number of times you may miss them." Thus, how the clinician asks these questions is important and can affect the overall relationship between the clinician and the patient [22]. Directly asking a patient about their views regarding medications can be very instructive [23,24]. It is important to avoid appearing punitive or authoritarian and to let the patient know that it is okay to disagree; the clinician should convey that they want to hear what the patient really thinks, not what he/she thinks the clinician wants to hear [10,23,24]. Flexibility in approach to treatment is required.

Additional tips include obtaining sufficient information before responding and to avoid jumping to conclusions [10]. When responding it will be important to not go beyond what the patient can accept for now. Even if there is disagreement about the need for medication, try to maintain and even strengthen the therapeutic alliance [23].

Interventions targeting nonadherence

The type of intervention will need to be matched to the cause of the partial or nonadherence but can be subdivided into "will not adhere" and "cannot adhere" [10]. If the adherence problem is that the patient "will not adhere," the intervention should focus on strengthening the patient's perceived benefits of medication and minimizing the patient's perceived costs, all within the context of a strong therapeutic alliance. Maximizing efficacy and tolerability involves a patient-specific selection of therapies. If the adherence problem is that the patient "cannot adhere," then addressing the barriers to adherence may be effective. These include the availability of pillboxes in locations that are easy to remember, self-monitoring tools such as checklists, establishment of routines, and the consideration of long-acting injectable antipsychotics [10]. More formal approaches have been studied including cognitive adaptation therapy that includes environmental supports to cue behavior [25].

Monitoring adherence

Research in adherence has used a number of measurement methods; however, none of them are perfect. Prescription fill rates at pharmacies, inspection of pill bottles, electronic counters embedded on medicine bottle caps, and similar measures do not necessarily reflect whether the medication is actually taken. Plasma levels of the prescribed medications can be helpful, although there is wide variation in levels for many of the medications in common use; moreover, the test can be considered intrusive.

In the clinic the most common method is asking the patient. Interview style, as previously discussed, is key in getting the most truthful answer possible. Asking if the medicines are producing any beneficial effects can be helpful; it can be very reassuring if the patient can articulate a benefit, but if there are no perceived benefits from the medication, then this may be a warning sign [2]. Likewise, it is important to also ask if the medications are causing any harm, such as feeling sleepy, slowed down, or dull, or associated with changes in weight, constipation, or sexual problems.

Alternate medication formulations

Liquid or orally disintegrating tablets can be helpful for patients with adherence problems (especially if the problems are related to swallowing pills); however, these formulations still need to be administered daily. Depot formulations can be administered every 2 weeks or every month, depending on the agent under consideration; yet, someone who is not responding adequately to an oral medication is unlikely to then respond to its depot formulation unless they were a nonresponder because of nonadherence. Potential advantages of depot antipsychotic formulations include the reduction of plasma level deviations [26] and elimination of guesswork about adherence status, thus helping to disentangle reasons for poor response to medication [27]. Depot formulations can help eliminate the abrupt loss of efficacy that can occur if oral doses are missed [26,27]. There is reduction in risk of relapse with the use of depot antipsychotics versus oral antipsychotics as demonstrated in long-term studies [28]. Many patients prefer them, especially if already receiving them [29]. Potential obstacles to depot antipsychotic formulations include lack of infrastructure in outpatient settings, acquisition costs, requirement for concomitant oral medications in addition to the depot injection, and anti-injection sentiments [26,27,30–32].

Summary

Partial and nonadherence is common in people being treated for chronic diseases, including schizophrenia. If unrecognized, lack of efficacy because of partial or nonadherence may lead to the mistaken impression of treatment-resistance to the medication being prescribed. Predictors of partial or nonadherence include a prior history of nonadherence, substance use, and alcohol use. The interview style and the therapeutic alliance are central for the accurate assessment of partial and/or nonadherence, and the appropriate implementation of intervention strategies.

References

1 Osterberg L, Blaschke T. Adherence to medication. *N Engl J Med*. 2005;353:487-497.

2 Velligan DI, Weiden PJ, Sajatovic M, et al. The expert consensus guideline series: adherence problems in patients with serious and persistent mental illness. *J Clin Psychiatry*. 2009;70(suppl 4):1-46.

3 Velligan DI, Wang M, Diamond P, et al. Relationships among subjective and objective measures of adherence to oral antipsychotic medications. *Psychiatr Serv*. 2007;58:1187-1192.

4 Velligan DI, Lam YW, Glahn DC, et al. Defining and assessing adherence to oral antipsychotics: a review of the literature. *Schizophr Bull*. 2006;32:724-742.

5 Valenstein M, Ganoczy D, McCarthy JF, Kim HM, Lee TA, Blow FC. Antipsychotic adherence over time among patients receiving treatment for schizophrenia: a retrospective review. *J Clin Psychiatry*. 2006;67:1542-1550.

6 Byerly MJ, Nakonezny PA, Lescouflair E. Antipsychotic medication adherence in schizophrenia. *Psychiatr Clin North Am*. 2007;30:437-452.

7 Perkins DO. Predictors of noncompliance in patients with schizophrenia. *J Clin Psychiatry.* 2002;63:1121-1128.

8 Lacro JP, Dunn LB, Dolder CR, Leckband SG, Jeste DV. Prevalence of and risk factors for medication nonadherence in patients with schizophrenia: a comprehensive review of recent literature. *J Clin Psychiatry.* 2002;63:892-909.

9 Weiden P, Rapkin B, Zygmunt A, Mott T, Goldman D, Frances A. Postdischarge medication compliance of inpatients converted from an oral to a depot neuroleptic regimen. *Psychiatr Serv.* 1995;46:1049-1054.

10 Weiden PJ. Understanding and addressing adherence issues in schizophrenia: from theory to practice. *J Clin Psychiatry.* 2007;68(suppl 14):14-19.

11 Frank AF, Gunderson JG. The role of the therapeutic alliance in the treatment of schizophrenia. Relationship to course and outcome. *Arch Gen Psychiatry.* 1990;47:228-236.

12 Lincoln TM, Lüllmann E, Rief W. Correlates and long-term consequences of poor insight in patients with schizophrenia. A systematic review. *Schizophr Bull.* 2007;33:1324-1342.

13 Citrome L. Treatment-refractory schizophrenia: what is it and what has been done about it? *Neuropsychiatry.* 2011;1:325-347.

14 Weiden PJ, Buckley PF. Reducing the burden of side effects during long-term antipsychotic therapy: the role of "switching" medications. *J Clin Psychiatry.* 2007;68(suppl 6):14-23.

15 Tandon R. Safety and tolerability: how do newer generation "atypical" antipsychotics compare? *Psychiatr Q.* 2002;73:297-311.

16 Ascher-Svanum H, Zhu B, Faries D, Lacro JP, Dolder CR. A prospective study of risk factors for nonadherence with antipsychotic medication in the treatment of schizophrenia. *J Clin Psychiatry.* 2006;67:1114-1123.

17 Regier DA, Farmer ME, Rae DS, et al. Comorbidity of mental disorders with alcohol and other drug abuse. Results from the Epidemiologic Catchment Area (ECA) Study. *JAMA.* 1990;264:2511-2518.

18 Lybrand J, Caroff S. Management of schizophrenia with substance use disorders. *Psychiatr Clin North Am.* 2009;32:821-833.

19 Lieberman JA, Stroup TS, McEvoy JP, et al; Clinical Antipsychotic Trials of Intervention Effectiveness (CATIE) Investigators. Effectiveness of antipsychotic drugs in patients with chronic schizophrenia. *N Engl J Med.* 2005;353:1209-1223.

20 Van Dorn RA, Desmarais SL, Scott Young M, Sellers BG, Swartz MS. Assessing illicit drug use among adults with schizophrenia. *Psychiatr Res.* 2012;200:228-236.

21 Kerfoot KE, Rosenheck RA, Petrakis IL, et al; CATIE Investigators. Substance use and schizophrenia: adverse correlates in the CATIE study sample. *Schizophr Res.* 2011;132:177-182.

22 Velligan DI, Weiden PJ, Sajatovic M, et al. Assessment of adherence problems in patients with serious and persistent mental illness: recommendations from the Expert Consensus Guidelines. *J Psychiatr Pract.* 2010;16:34-45.

23 Weiden PJ. Why did John Nash stop his medication? *J Psychiatr Pract.* 2002;8:386-392.

24 McCabe R, Heath C, Burns T, Priebe S. Engagement of patients with psychosis in the consultation: conversation analytic study. *BMJ.* 2002;325:1148-1151.

25 Velligan D, Diamond PM, Mintz J, et al. The use of individually tailored environmental supports to improve medication adherence and outcomes in schizophrenia. *Schizophr Bull.* 2008;34:483-493.

26 McEvoy JP. Risks versus benefits of different types of long-acting injectable antipsychotics. *J Clin Psychiatry.* 2006;67(suppl 5):15-18.

27 Kane JM, Leucht S, Carpenter D, Docherty JP. Optimizing pharmacologic treatment of psychotic disorders. Introduction: methods, commentary, and summary. *J Clin Psychiatry.* 2003;64(suppl 12):5-19.

28 Leucht C, Heres S, Kane JM et al. Oral versus depot antipsychotic drugs for schizophrenia - a critical systematic review and meta-analysis of randomised long-term trials. *Schizophr Res.* 2011;127:83-92.

29 Patel MX, De Zoysa N, Baker D, David AS. Antipsychotic depot medication and attitudes of community psychiatric nurses. *J Psychiatr Ment Health Nurs*. 2005;12:237-244.

30 Citrome L. Patient perspectives in the development and use of long-acting antipsychotics in schizophrenia: focus on olanzapine long-acting injection. *Patient Prefer Adherence*. 2009;3:345-355.

31 Citrome L. Paliperidone palmitate – review of the efficacy, safety and cost of a new second-generation depot antipsychotic medication. *Int J Clin Pract*. 2010;64:216-239.

32 Citrome L, Levine J, Allingham B. Utilization of depot neuroleptic medication in psychiatric inpatients. *Psychopharmacol Bull*. 1996;32:321-326.

Chapter 4

Dosing of antipsychotics – what evidence do we use?

Practice-based evidence

One method of determining potentially useful antipsychotic dosing ranges is to examine what is being used in the field. Once a medication has become available for some time and clinicians are experienced in using it, a possible assumption is that the doses used in the "real world" may be the best ones to try. For patients with a suboptimal treatment response, a place to look for dosing information would be among inpatients with persistent symptoms.

The average daily dose of selected antipsychotics were examined in a report on antipsychotic dosing for patients hospitalized for intermediate- and long-term care [1]. In 2003, the average daily dose of risperidone (4.5 mg) was much lower than 16 mg/day, the US Food and Drug Administration (FDA)-approved maximum dose as indicated in the product labeling. In contrast to risperidone, the average daily dose of olanzapine (22.5 mg) was higher than the FDA-approved product label maximum of 20 mg/day. A possible reason for the lower average daily dose of risperidone is the likelihood that an increase in risperidone dose does not necessarily lead to an increase in therapeutic response but increases the risk of extrapyramidal symptoms. The higher average daily dose of olanzapine may be due to the possibility that for some patients an increase in dose leads to an increase in therapeutic response that possibly extends beyond 20 mg/day [1]. Later reports from the New York State Office of Mental Health focused on dosing of quetiapine [2] and ziprasidone [3]. For both quetiapine and ziprasidone, the average daily dose increased over

L. Citrome, *Handbook of Treatment-resistant Schizophrenia*,
DOI: 10.1007/978-1-908517-88-3_4,
© Springer Healthcare 2013

time and in 2004 about one-third of people prescribed quetiapine were receiving a dose in excess of 750 mg/day [2]. In 2006, over half of people prescribed ziprasidone were receiving a dose in excess of 160 mg/day [3]. Over this period of time, the average daily dose of aripiprazole declined, with approximately only 10% receiving a dose in excess of 30 mg/day [4]. Practice-based evidence thus suggests that higher doses of olanzapine, quetiapine, and ziprasidone may be helpful for more difficult-to-treat patients, but that this may not be the case for risperidone or aripiprazole where high dosing does not appear to be commonly used. Fixed-dose, randomized, double-blind clinical trials of the antipsychotic in question, specifically designed to delineate therapeutic dose–response relationships, are needed to confirm a dose–response beyond on-label doses [5].

The newer second-generation antipsychotics iloperidone, asenapine, and lurasidone have only recently been introduced [6], and thus no relevant practice-based dosing data for these agents are available at this time.

Research-based evidence

Initial dosing recommendations provided in product labeling are the result of carefully designed registration studies. These studies are focused on detecting a signal of efficacy for the test drug compared with placebo. The inclusion and exclusion criteria for these studies are carefully designed to disallow participation by patients who may be treatment-refractory, are actively using alcohol or substances, have significant somatic health problems, or are unable to provide written informed consent. These exclusions impact on the generalizability of the results and dosing recommendations, and its applicability in the clinic setting.

There have been few double-blind clinical trials that have tested doses of olanzapine greater than 20 mg/day, but the trials do suggest that these doses may be helpful in selected patients who are treatment-resistant, have high levels of psychopathology, or who are acutely agitated [7]. In a flexible-dose, 14-week, double-blind, randomized study of 157 patients with schizophrenia and suboptimal treatment response, the overall pattern of results was that clozapine and olanzapine had similar general antipsychotic efficacy; the mean dose achieved for olanzapine was approximately 30 mg/day [8]. In order to ascertain the presence or absence of a therapeutic dose response for olanzapine that extends beyond 20 mg/day, the manufacturer conducted a randomized, double-blind, 8-week, fixed-dose study comparing olanzapine 10, 20, and 40 mg/day in 599 patients with schizophrenia or schizoaffective disorder and suboptimal response to current treatment [9]. All dose groups showed statistically significant improvement in Positive and Negative Syndrome Scale (PANSS) total scores from baseline to endpoint without a significant dose–response relationship. However, a post-hoc analysis of response demonstrated better response at higher doses for patients with higher baseline PANSS scores. On a cautionary note, there was a significant dose response for the adverse events of a mean increase in body weight and a mean increase in prolactin levels [9].

Two double-blind, randomized clinical trials have tested above-label doses of quetiapine; neither trial supported doses in excess of 600–800 mg/day [10,11]. In one of the studies, participants were patients with schizophrenia or schizoaffective disorder hospitalized at two state-operated psychiatric facilities in New York [10]. In order to be eligible for randomization, patients were required to prospectively fail to demonstrate an initial therapeutic response during a 4-week run-in phase with quetiapine at 600 mg/day. Patients were then randomized to either continue quetiapine at 600 mg/day for an additional 8 weeks or to receive 1200 mg/day quetiapine instead. No significant differences were observed between the high dose ($n = 29$) and standard dose ($n = 31$) groups in mean change in PANSS total score. The second study, conducted at multiple sites in Canada, compared quetiapine 1200 mg/day with 800 mg/day [11]. Subjects were required to prospectively fail to demonstrate an adequate therapeutic response during a 4-week run-in phase with quetiapine titrated to 800 mg/day. Again, no advantages were evident for quetiapine outside the approved dose range.

Ziprasidone 320 mg/day was compared with 160 mg/day in an 8-week, double-blind, randomized, multicenter study conducted in the United States [12]. Patients were required to have persistent psychotic symptoms despite being treated with ziprasidone 160 mg/day for a minimum of 3 weeks. The two treatment groups did not differ in their response during the 8-week trial on any clinical rating.

Thus, research-based evidence has largely failed to support the high dosing of those antipsychotics that are routinely prescribed in that manner in clinical practice, with the possible exception of some subpopulations of patients being treated with high doses of olanzapine.

Reconciling doses used in clinical practice with those supported by clinical research

Given the general lack of supporting research evidence for the high doses of antipsychotics that are often prescribed, a discussion of the limitations of clinical trials is in order. Clinical trials can answer questions about potential major differences that can exist between groups of patients; however, there may be large differences that can be observed in how an individual has responded to any particular intervention. The clinician treating an individual may be inclined to push a dose higher, provided that the medication is reasonably tolerable and that the patient is willing to adhere to it. Yet, the lack of confirmatory controlled clinical trial evidence supporting most instances of high dosing is not reassuring.

Dosing may be confounded by pharmacokinetic issues that can interfere with achieving adequate plasma levels [13–15]. For example, carbamazepine or rifampin can induce the CYP3A4 enzyme system and result in subtherapeutic antipsychotic levels for those agents metabolized through that system. Cigarette smoking also may have this effect for drugs metabolized through the CYP1A2 enzyme system; lowered clozapine or olanzapine plasma levels have been observed in patients who resume smoking after being discharged from a nonsmoking inpatient environment. Rapid metabolizers through CYP2D6 can also interfere with achieving therapeutic levels of some agents. Inhibitors of CYP enzyme systems can also lead to issues in terms of excessive plasma levels. Some antipsychotics, such as ziprasidone and lurasidone, must be taken with food (500 calories and 350 calories, respectively) in order to have sufficient bioavailability [16].

Summary

In addition to partial or nonadherence, inadequate antipsychotic dosing may confound the assessment of patients with treatment-resistance. It is common clinical practice to increase antipsychotic dosing in the face of inadequate response; however, the research evidence that supports going above the maximum recommended dose is often lacking. Pharmacokinetic issues may further complicate matters with drug–drug interactions sometimes having a profound effect on antipsychotic plasma levels and can potentially alter antipsychotic efficacy or tolerability.

References

1 Citrome L, Jaffe A, Levine J. Dosing of second-generation antipsychotic medication in a state hospital system. *J Clin Psychopharmacol*. 2005;25:388-391.

2 Citrome L, Jaffe A, Levine J, Lindenmayer JP. Dosing of quetiapine in schizophrenia: how clinical practice differs from registration studies. *J Clin Psychiatry*. 2005;66:1512-1516.

3 Citrome L, Jaffe A, Levine J. How dosing of ziprasidone in a state hospital system differs from product labeling. *J Clin Psychiatry*. 2009;70:975-982.

4 Citrome L, Jaffe A, Levine J. Datapoints: The ups and downs of dosing second-generation antipsychotics. *Psychiatr Serv*. 2007;58:11.

5 Citrome L, Volavka J. Optimal dosing of atypical antipsychotics in adults: a review of the current evidence. *Harv Rev Psychiatry*. 2002;10:280-291.

6 Citrome L. Iloperidone, asenapine, and lurasidone: a brief overview of 3 new second-generation antipsychotics. *Postgrad Med*. 2011;123:153-162.

7 Citrome L, Kantrowitz JT. Olanzapine dosing above the licensed range is more efficacious than lower doses: fact or fiction? *Expert Rev Neurother*. 2009;9:1045-1058.

8 Volavka J, Czobor P, Sheitman B, et al. Clozapine, olanzapine, risperidone, and haloperidol in the treatment of patients with chronic schizophrenia and schizoaffective disorder. *Am J Psychiatry*. 2002;159:255-262.

9 Kinon BJ, Volavka J, Stauffer V, et al. Standard and higher dose of olanzapine in patients with schizophrenia or schizoaffective disorder: a randomized, double-blind, fixed-dose study. *J Clin Psychopharmacol*. 2008;28:392-400.

10 Lindenmayer JP, Citrome L, Khan A, Kaushik S, Kaushik S. A randomized, double-blind, parallel-group, fixed-dose, clinical trial of quetiapine at 600 versus 1200 mg/d for patients with treatment-resistant schizophrenia or schizoaffective disorder. *J Clin Psychopharmacol*. 2011;31:160-168.

11 Honer WG, MacEwan GW, Gendron A, et al; STACK Study Group. A randomized, double-blind, placebo-controlled study of the safety and tolerability of high-dose quetiapine in patients with persistent symptoms of schizophrenia or schizoaffective disorder. *J Clin Psychiatry*. 2012;73:13-20.

12 Goff D, McEvoy J, Citrome L, et al. High-dose oral ziprasidone versus conventional dosing in schizophrenia patients with residual symptoms: the ZEBRAS study. *J Clin Psychopharmacol*. In press.

13 Preskorn SH. Clinically important differences in the pharmacokinetics of the ten newer "atypical" antipsychotics: part 1. *J Psychiatr Pract*. 2012;18:199-204.

14 Preskorn SH. Clinically important differences in the pharmacokinetics of the ten newer "atypical" antipsychotics: part 2. Metabolism and elimination. *J Psychiatr Pract*. 2012;18:361-368.

15 Preskorn SH. Clinically important differences in the pharmacokinetics of the ten newer "atypical" antipsychotics: part 3. Effects of renal and hepatic impairment. *J Psychiatr Pract*. 2012;18:430-437.

16 Citrome L. Lurasidone in schizophrenia: new information about dosage and place in therapy. *Adv Ther*. 2012;29:815-825.

PART TWO

Management approaches

Chapter 5

Psychopharmacological approaches

Overview

Randomized clinical trials in patients with treatment-resistant schizophrenia have tested antipsychotic monotherapies, antipsychotic combination therapies, and nonantipsychotic augmentation strategies. Clozapine has been a landmark medication for patients with treatment-resistant schizophrenia, but attempts to specifically augment it have not resulted in any further breakthroughs of the same magnitude. Logical candidates for antipsychotic augmentation have in general not been successful, including anticholinesterase inhibitors and other agents used to treat cognitive decline in Alzheimer's disease. Antipsychotic combinations have resulted in incremental improvements at best. Research being done with antidepressant medications and with agents that impact the glutamate receptor hold the greatest promise at this time [1].

Heterogeneity of antipsychotics

There is extensive heterogeneity among first- and second-generation antipsychotics as well as overlaps between them in terms of their effects [2]. It would not be unreasonable to prescribe a different antipsychotic from either class if faced with a patient who has not adequately responded to their initial antipsychotic; however, the largest differences between first-line antipsychotics may be in terms of safety and tolerability. For example, first-generation antipsychotics usually elicit more extrapyramidal adverse events and possible tardive dyskinesia as well as elevations in

L. Citrome, *Handbook of Treatment-resistant Schizophrenia*,
DOI: 10.1007/978-1-908517-88-3_5,
© Springer Healthcare 2013

prolactin levels than most second-generation antipsychotics. In contrast, some second-generation antipsychotics tend to be associated with more weight gain and disturbances in lipid and glucose regulation than first-generation antipsychotics. Yet, there are again considerable differences between individual agents in each class and overlaps between the two groups in terms of side effects. For example, elevated prolactin levels can be observed with risperidone, and weight gain and metabolic disturbances can be observed with chlorpromazine. It is thought that these differences among the antipsychotics are due to their unique receptor-binding affinity profiles. In addition, people with schizophrenia also form a heterogeneous group with different biological vulnerabilities. In general, the treatment selection for a patient should focus on the suitability of an individual antipsychotic for that patient rather than on the group or class of the drug.

Although first-generation antipsychotics are inexpensive and the availability of depot versions of some first-generation antipsychotics can make their choice compelling, extrapyramidal symptoms are not benign. Extrapyramidal symptoms have been identified as a risk factor for the future development of tardive dyskinesia [3]. Moreover, treatment of extrapyramidal symptoms with anticholinergic agents such as benztropine can further impair cognitive functioning [4].

Evidence base for antipsychotic monotherapies

Antipsychotic monotherapy would be the simplest regimen to implement, assuming that the dose is optimized and adherence can be anticipated. A series of meta-analyses of antipsychotic efficacy have been conducted suggesting that there are three "tiers" of antipsychotic medications, as measured by their ability to reduce the symptoms of schizophrenia [5–7]. Clozapine is the sole member of the first tier, evidencing the largest effect size difference when compared with first-generation antipsychotics. In the second tier are olanzapine, risperidone and amisulpride, which although also demonstrate effect size differences when compared with first-generation antipsychotics, these differences are not as large as observed with clozapine. The remaining second-generation antipsychotics are in the third tier, together with first-generation antipsychotics; although the agents in the third tier have differing tolerability profiles, they have similar overall efficacy [5–7]. Although not included in these meta-analyses, it is note-worthy that depot formulations for risperidone and olanzapine are available. Also missing from these meta-analyses are the three more recently approved second-generation antipsychotics iloperidone, asenapine, and lurasidone [8]. Their relative efficacy compared with each other or versus other antipsychotics has not yet been tested either directly in well-controlled and adequately powered randomized clinical trials or indirectly through meta-analyses. A general caveat is that these meta-analyses focused on efficacy and derived their findings from controlled clinical trials. In clinical practice, tolerability differences between the agents may greatly influence treatment selection for the individual patient who may or may not be particularly vulnerable to the adverse events in question.

Clozapine's advantages over risperidone and quetiapine (but not olanzapine) were also statistically significant and clinically relevant in an effectiveness study, as measured by time to all-cause discontinuation [9]. Consistent results in favor of clozapine (and olanzapine) had been obtained in a prior randomized controlled trial that compared clozapine, olanzapine, risperidone, and haloperidol over a 14-week period, using the Positive and Negative Syndrome Scale (PANSS) to measure efficacy [10].

Table 5.1 lists several studies of antipsychotic monotherapies for treatment-resistant schizophrenia [1,9–39]. Although most of the studies are for adult patients, there are also studies that have examined childhood-onset treatment-refractory schizophrenia [14,33,35]. In most studies, clozapine consistently demonstrated superiority over comparators. In addition to clozapine being efficacious in treatment-resistant schizophrenia, clozapine is US Food and Drug Administration (FDA)-approved for the indication of reduction in the risk of recurrent suicidal behavior in schizophrenia or schizoaffective disorder [40]. Clozapine has also demonstrated superiority over other agents in the reduction of aggression, although it has not received regulatory approval for this indication [41]. In treatment-naïve first-episode schizophrenia, clozapine has been shown to be more effective than chlorpromazine in terms of time to remission and maintenance of remission [42]. Despite these clear advantages, there is considerable tolerability and safety challenges involved when prescribing clozapine, relegating this agent to second-line status [43].

Randomized controlled trials of antipsychotic monotherapy in treatment-refractory schizophrenia

Author and year	Study duration (weeks)	Number randomized	Antipsychotic	Efficacy*
Kane 1988 [11]	6	268	Clozapine	Clozapine > chlorpromazine
Pickar 1992 [12]	Varied	21	Clozapine	Clozapine > fluphenazine or placebo
Breier 1994 [13]	10	39	Clozapine	Clozapine > haloperidol
Kumra 1996 [14]	6	21 children	Clozapine	Clozapine > haloperidol
Hong 1997 [15]	12	40	Clozapine	Clozapine > chlorpromazine
Rosenheck 1997 [16]	1 year	423	Clozapine	Clozapine > haloperidol
Buchanan 1998 [17]	10	75	Clozapine	Clozapine > haloperidol
Kane 2001 [18]	29	71	Clozapine	Clozapine > haloperidol
Volavka 2002 [10]	14	157	Clozapine, olanzapine or risperidone	Clozapine ~ olanzapine > risperidone > haloperidol
McEvoy 2006 [9]	NA	99	Clozapine	Clozapine ~ olanzapine > risperidone, quetiapine
Bondolfi 1998 [19]	8	86	Risperidone	Risperidone ~ clozapine
Wirshing 1999 [20]	8	67	Risperidone	Risperidone > haloperidol (at 4 weeks but not 8 weeks)
Breier 1999 [21]	6	29	Risperidone	Risperidone < clozapine
Wahlbeck 2000 [22]	10	19	Risperidone	Risperidone ~ clozapine
Azorin 2001 [23]	12	273	Risperidone	Risperidone < clozapine
Zhang 2001 [24]	12	78	Risperidone	Risperidone > haloperidol
Liberman 2002 [25]	8	36	Risperidone	Risperidone ~ haloperidol
Conley 2005 [26]	12	38	Risperidone or quetiapine	Risperidone ~ quetiapine ~ fluphenazine
Conley 1998 [27]	6	84	Olanzapine	Olanzapine ~ chlorpromazine
Breier 1999 [28]	6	526	Olanzapine	Olanzapine > haloperidol
Tollefson 2001 [29]	18	180	Olanzapine	Olanzapine ~ clozapine
Conley 2003 [30]	16	13	Olanzapine	Olanzapine < clozapine
Bitter 2004 [31]	18	147	Olanzapine	Olanzapine ~ clozapine

Table 5.1 Randomized controlled trials of antipsychotic monotherapy in treatment-refractory schizophrenia (continues opposite).

Author and year	Study duration (weeks)	Number randomized	Antipsychotic	Efficacy*
Buchanan 2005 [32]	16	63	Olanzapine	Olanzapine ~ haloperidol
Shaw 2006 [33]	8	25 children	Olanzapine	Olanzapine < clozapine
Meltzer 2008 [34]	6 months	40	Olanzapine	Olanzapine ~ clozapine
Kumra 2008 [35]	12	39 children	Olanzapine	Olanzapine < clozapine
Emsley 2000 [36]	8	288	Quetiapine	Quetiapine > haloperidol
Kane 2006 [37]	12	306	Ziprasidone	Ziprasidone > chlorpromazine
Sacchetti 2009 [38]	18	147	Ziprasidone	Ziprasidone ~ clozapine
Kane 2007 [39]	6	300	Aripiprazole	Aripiprazole ~ perphenazine

Table 5.1 Randomized controlled trials of antipsychotic monotherapy in treatment-refractory schizophrenia (continued). All studies enrolled adults unless otherwise noted. *In some studies, multiple different outcomes were measured and some small differences may have emerged that are different from the overall results as noted here. ~, similar to or no difference from. Reproduced with permission from Citrome [1].

Clozapine use is associated with leukopenia and agranulocytosis, thus frequent white blood cell count monitoring is required. One study found that the risk of drug-induced blood dyscrasias appears to be higher at the start of treatment and then decreases from 0.70/1000 patient-years in the second 6 months of treatment to 0.39/1000 patient-years after the first year [44]. Prior to starting clozapine treatment, FDA guidelines require that the patient's white blood cell count must be at least 3500 mm^3 and the absolute neutrophil count must be at least 2000 mm^3. For the first 6 months, patients receiving clozapine must have a weekly blood test for white blood cell count and absolute neutrophil count [45]. The dispensing pharmacist must have the blood work result prior to releasing the drug to the patient; the blood draw date must be within the previous 7 days for the pharmacist to dispense a 1-week supply of clozapine. After 6 months of continuous therapy with clozapine without any interruptions because of a low white blood cell count and/or absolute neutrophil count (defined as a white blood cell count <3000 mm^3 and/or absolute neutrophil count <1500 mm^3 or increased monitoring [when white blood cell count <3500 mm^3 and/or absolute neutrophil count <2000 mm^3])

the patient's blood monitoring may be done every 14 days and a 2-week supply of clozapine can be dispensed. After 12 months of continuous clozapine therapy (6 months of continuous weekly monitoring, then 6 months of continuous biweekly monitoring) without any interruptions or increased monitoring, the patient may have blood monitoring done every 4 weeks and can receive a 4-week supply of clozapine [45]. A potential benefit of these monitoring requirements is that the increased frequency of visits can be used to foster greater patient engagement with treatment and promote a stronger therapeutic alliance. Peer-led clozapine support groups, available in some communities, can help facilitate adherence to monitoring requirements.

Although the recommended target dose for clozapine is 300–450 mg/day, some patients may only tolerate a lower dose. For cigarette smokers, the induction of the CYP1A2 enzyme system may require higher doses. Obtaining a plasma level may be helpful if an adequate response is not achieved, despite presumed good adherence [46]. Plasma levels equal or greater to 350 ng/mL constitute an optimal clozapine trial. Because of tolerability concerns, including the potential for dose-related seizures and orthostatic hypotension, slow and careful titration of clozapine is necessary, making clozapine monotherapy a less than ideal choice for antipsychotic treatment if rapid control of acute psychotic symptoms is required. In terms of monitoring for adverse effects, clozapine's product information carries additional warnings about myocarditis (difficult to diagnose and commonly used tests have limited sensitivity) and increased mortality in elderly patients with dementia-related psychosis. Common side effects (frequency) include hypersalivation (31–48%), excessive sedation (39–46%), weight gain (4–31%) or metabolic abnormalities, tachycardia (25%), dizziness (19–27%), and constipation (14–25%) [45]. Since constipation can be potentially severe and life-threatening, many clinicians prescribe prophylactic stool softeners to patients on clozapine and prone to this adverse event [45]. The ethnicity of the patient may influence the risk of adverse effects, as observed in a study of aggressive inpatients where African Americans receiving clozapine were more likely to develop metabolic abnormalities than patients in other ethnic groups [47]. Patients placed on clozapine require careful monitoring for metabolic adverse effects and the use of remediative psychosocial, lifestyle, and adjunctive medication interventions (such as statins) when necessary [48].

However, not all patients with treatment-resistant schizophrenia can tolerate clozapine or are willing to have their blood monitored as required, so other second-generation antipsychotics have been suggested as possible substitutes for clozapine. Olanzapine has established superior efficacy to first-generation antipsychotics [5–7] and was perhaps comparable to clozapine in some studies [9,10,29,31,34]. Although risperidone also appears to be comparable to clozapine in some studies [19,22], the superiority of clozapine was evident in others [9,21,23], and thus the evidence is more consistently in favor of olanzapine in treatment-refractory schizophrenia rather than using risperidone in this population. Favorable results were also observed for ziprasidone compared with clozapine in a randomized clinical trial [38], but patients enrolled in that study were not necessarily treatment-resistant in terms of efficacy and may have been primarily intolerant to prior treatments; the study design required them to be resistant and/or intolerant to at least three cycles of different treatments prior to randomization. Similar imprecision in inclusion requirements also affects the interpretation of a study comparing olanzapine and clozapine [31] and another study comparing risperidone with clozapine [19]. In general, efficacy differences between the antipsychotic groups in these studies are often small and are overshadowed by the potentially large individual differences in response that can be observed in clinical practice.

An important agent in the early history of the psychopharmacology of schizophrenia is reserpine, an antihypertensive medication that had been used as an antipsychotic. It is thought to deplete monoamine neurotransmitters, including dopamine. There are no available reports of a randomized controlled study of reserpine specifically for treatment-resistant schizophrenia, and the agent is often forgotten. A review of the use of reserpine in schizophrenia is available that summarizes the available controlled studies for reserpine for psychosis [49]. The studies were conducted more than 50 years ago using the standards for such trials as they existed at that time. There is anecdotal and uncontrolled evidence that some patients who respond poorly to "neuroleptics" may improve with reserpine. Trials of reserpine may be warranted in some treatment-resistant patients, but adverse events such as severe depression, significant hypotension, exacerbation of asthma, peptic ulceration and hemorrhage, and extrapyramidal symptoms can be problematic. There is evidence that a gradual increase to a full dose reduces some side effects.

Evidence base for antipsychotic combination therapy

In the quest of achieving better efficacy, combinations of antipsychotics are commonly used when managing chronically ill people with schizophrenia. In state-operated psychiatric hospitals in New York, about half of all patients receive more than one antipsychotic [50], and at doses that are not any lower than what would ordinarily be used in monotherapy [51]. Unfortunately, the evidence base supporting this approach is very limited, thus the practice-based evidence of high utilization of combinations of antipsychotics is not consistent with the available research-based evidence.

Table 5.2 lists several studies of antipsychotic combination therapy for treatment-resistant schizophrenia [1,52–70]. These trials generally enrolled patients who had a prior inadequate therapeutic response to clozapine monotherapy [1]. There are few individual studies that unequivocally support the use of antipsychotic combination treatment

Author and year	Study duration (weeks)	Number randomized	Combination	Efficacy*
Potter 1989 [52]	8	57	Chlorpromazine and clozapine	Chlorpromazine and clozapine ~ or > clozapine or chlorpromazine
Shiloh 1997 [53]	10	28	Sulpiride and clozapine	Sulpiride and clozapine > clozapine
Josiassen 2005 [54]	12	40	Risperidone and clozapine	Risperidone and clozapine > clozapine
Anil Yağcioğlu 2005 [55]	6	30	Risperidone and clozapine	Risperidone and clozapine < clozapine

Table 5.2 Randomized controlled trials of antipsychotic combination therapies in treatment-refractory schizophrenia (continues opposite).

Randomized controlled trials of antipsychotic combination therapies in treatment-refractory schizophrenia (continued)

Author and year	Study duration (weeks)	Number randomized	Combination	Efficacy*
Honer 2006 [56]	8	68	Risperidone and clozapine	Risperidone and clozapine ~ clozapine
Freudenreich 2007 [57]	6	24	Risperidone and clozapine	Risperidone and clozapine ~ or > clozapine
Weiner 2010 [58]	16	69	Risperidone and clozapine	Risperidone and clozapine ~ or > clozapine
Kreinin 2006 [59]	7	20	Amisulpride and clozapine	Amisulpride and clozapine ~ or > clozapine
Assion 2008 [60]	6	16	Amisulpride and clozapine	Amisulpride and clozapine ~ or > clozapine
Genç 2007 [61]	8	56	Amisulpride and clozapine	Amisulpride and clozapine > quetiapine and clozapine
Chang 2008 [62]	8	62	Aripiprazole and clozapine	Aripiprazole and clozapine ~ or > clozapine
Fleischhacker 2010 [63]	16	207	Aripiprazole and clozapine	Aripiprazole and clozapine ~ or > clozapine
Muscatello 2011 [64]	24	40	Aripiprazole and clozapine	Aripiprazole and clozapine > clozapine
Zink 2009 [65]	6	24	Ziprasidone and clozapine	Ziprasidone and clozapine ~ clozapine and risperidone
Kane 2009 [66]	16	323	Risperidone or quetiapine and aripiprazole	Risperidone or quetiapine and aripiprazole ~ risperidone or quetiapine
Henderson 2009 [67]	10	15	Aripiprazole and olanzapine	Aripiprazole and olanzapine ~ olanzapine
Shafti 2009 [68]	12	28	Fluphenazine decanoate and olanzapine	Fluphenazine decanoate and olanzapine ~ or > olanzapine
Kotler 2004 [69]	8	17	Sulpiride and olanzapine	Sulpiride and olanzapine ~ or > olanzapine
Takahashi 1999 [70]	8	24	Risperidone or mosapramine and one or more first-generation antipsychotics	Risperidone or mosapramine and one or more first-generation antipsychotics > one or more first-generation antipsychotics

Table 5.2 Randomized controlled trials of antipsychotic combination therapies in treatment-refractory schizophrenia (continued). As tested in randomized controlled trials; all studies enrolled adults. *In some studies, multiple different outcomes were measured and small advantages may be apparent; this is noted as ~ or >. ~, similar to or no difference from. Reproduced with permission from Citrome [1].

[53,54,61,64,70]; these include one trial of adjunctive sulpiride [53], one trial of adjunctive amisulpride or quetiapine (adjunctive amisulpride performed better than adjunctive quetiapine) [61], one trial of adjunctive risperidone [54], one trial of adjunctive risperidone or adjunctive mosapramine (adjunctive risperidone performed essentially the same as adjunctive mosapramine) [70], and one trial of adjunctive aripiprazole [64]. Sulpiride, amisulpride, and mosapramine are not available in the United States.

For the most commonly studied combinations, such as clozapine and risperidone, several negative or equivocal studies have also been published [55–58]. As noted in a Cochrane systematic review [71], study design issues, such as small sample size as well as the heterogeneity of comparisons, make it difficult to determine which antipsychotic is the best choice to add to clozapine. In their summary, the authors noted that, "When people on clozapine plus risperidone were compared to those on clozapine plus sulpiride, more people taking risperidone showed an improvement generally. However, when specific symptoms of schizophrenia were studied, there was change for the better in all groups but no second antipsychotic was significantly better than the one it was compared to. When looking at adverse effects, people taking sulpiride were slightly more likely to suffer from hypersalivation and weight gain than those risperidone." The authors continued, "Although there is a suggestion that adding a second antipsychotic may improve general functioning and decrease the symptoms of schizophrenia, it is still not possible to say which antipsychotic would help the most."

The overall effect size for a benefit with antipsychotic combinations is small, as noted in a meta-analysis of 14 studies (734 subjects) of clozapine with a second antipsychotic [72]. However, it is important to remember that there will always be individuals who appear to derive substantial therapeutic benefit from combination therapy even though this potentially large treatment effect cannot be easily demonstrated when comparing groups of patients in randomized controlled trials. The large observed heterogeneity in treatment response allows some degree of cautious optimism.

Evidence base for adjunctive nonantipsychotic medications

In addition to antipsychotic combination therapy, augmentation strategies with nonantipsychotic medications are also commonly used when treating patients with schizophrenia. Antidepressants, anticonvulsants and lithium are commonly used together with antipsychotics in patients with schizophrenia, although this use is "off-label."

For example, lithium and anticonvulsants are used in about half of all patients with schizophrenia hospitalized in facilities operated by the State of New York Office of Mental Health [73,74]. In 1998, valproate was the most commonly coprescribed mood stabilizer (and continues to be) with 35% of patients prescribed this agent. Notably, valproate use was neither brief nor prescribed at low doses; on average, patients received valproate for about two-thirds of their hospital stay at a mean dose of 1520 mg/day [73]. Impulsivity and hostility/aggression are often given as reasons for prescribing adjunctive lithium and anticonvulsants [75]. Unfortunately, early reports of benefit with adjunctive lithium and anticonvulsants in patients with schizophrenia have been negated by larger randomized controlled trials conducted later in the hopes of eventually obtaining regulatory approval [76]. Many of the early anecdotal reports were of patients with treatment-resistant schizophrenia but few controlled trials conducted later included this population. Of all of these "mood stabilizers," lamotrigine may be the most promising for treatment-resistant schizophrenia. In a meta-analysis specifically examining patients on clozapine who had been randomized to receive either adjunctive lamotrigine or adjunctive placebo, lamotrigine was superior to placebo augmentation in total score for symptoms of psychosis and scores for positive and negative symptoms [77]. Regarding the specific utility of anticonvulsants such as valproate to help manage persistent aggressive behavior, there is very limited information from controlled clinical trials [76]. In one 8-week, open-label trial in hospitalized patients with schizophrenia and hostile behavior, 33 patients were randomly assigned to receive either risperidone monotherapy or risperidone plus valproate [78]; although patients receiving combination therapy were more likely to complete the study, the investigators were unable to detect a meaningful advantage for combination therapy as measured by rating scales. It is important to keep in mind that aggression and violent behavior is multifactorial in etiology, and in patients with schizophrenia aggression can be driven by psychosis, impaired impulse control or personality disorder; as such, effective interventions will vary [79,80]. A more complete discussion of the assessment and management of aggression in schizophrenia can be found elsewhere [79–83].

Adjunctive antidepressant use is also common among patients being treated for schizophrenia [84], although they are less widely used in Asia compared to Western countries [85]. Antidepressants may be helpful in reducing depressive symptoms as well as negative symptoms in patients with schizophrenia; both depressive symptoms and negative symptoms are common and readily assessed, and reflect that schizophrenia is a complex multidimensional disorder [86,87]. About 40 randomized controlled trials have tested adjunctive antidepressants in patients with chronic schizophrenia for ongoing depressive symptoms and/or negative symptoms; the agents studied included tricyclic and tetracyclic antidepressants, serotonin-specific reuptake inhibitors, monoamine oxidase inhibitors, mirtazapine, reboxetine, ritanserin, and trazodone [1]. Not all of the agents tested are commercially available in every country. In a meta-analysis of 23 trials of the effect of antidepressants on the negative symptoms of chronic schizophrenia, the authors concluded that antidepressants when combined with antipsychotics were more effective in treating the negative symptoms of schizophrenia than antipsychotics alone, as measured by the standardized mean difference between end-of-trial and baseline scores of negative symptoms [88]. A subgroup analysis revealed significant responses for fluoxetine, trazodone, and ritanserin.

The treatment domain of cognition has been a source of active interest. There have been more than 50 randomized controlled trials of agents that are thought to be potentially useful in ameliorating cognitive dysfunction in patients with chronic schizophrenia [1]. Unfortunately, clinical trials with commercially available logical candidate agents, such as donepezil, galantamine, memantine, rivastigmine, methylphenidate, guanfacine, atomoxetine, modafinil, and armodafinil (medications used to manage Alzheimer's disease, attention-deficit hyperactivity disorder, and daytime alertness), have not yielded encouraging results.

Other experimental approaches to augment antipsychotic medication in patients with chronic schizophrenia have included acetylsalicylic acid, nonsteroidal anti-inflammatory agents, antiglucocorticoids, beta blockers (for persistent aggressive behavior in particular), GABA-A receptor drugs (tested for cognition), neurosteroids and hormones, omega-3 fatty acids, opioids, peptides, purinergic agents, serotonin 5-HT$_{1A}$ receptor agonists, serotonin 5-HT$_3$ receptor antagonists, and complementary/alternative medicines (ginkgo, Yi-gan san, megavitamins). Preliminary promising results (≥ 2 positive studies and ≤ 2 negative studies) have emerged from studies of celecoxib, neurosteroids and hormones, purinergic agents, serotonin 5-HT$_{1A}$ receptor agonists, and serotonin 5-HT$_3$ receptor antagonists [1]. Potential benefits have also been noted for agents that target the alpha-7 nicotinic receptor [89,90]. Experimental agents that act on glutamate receptors are garnering intense interest with commercial drug developers, and are discussed in greater detail below regarding their potential in ameliorating negative symptoms and cognitive impairment.

Glutamate receptors as a therapeutic target

There is substantial research activity in the area of schizophrenia and the glutamate neurotransmitter system, with some glutamatergic drugs having reached Phase III in clinical development [91]. The interplay between glutamate and dopamine may provide a way to develop therapeutic agents that could treat the negative and cognitive symptoms of schizophrenia. The mechanism of action of these agents involves consideration of the *N*-methyl-d-aspartate (NMDA) receptor hypofunction hypothesis [91]. Under normal circumstances, the NMDA receptor, activated by glutamate, helps regulate the mesolimbic dopamine pathway by tonic inhibition of dopamine neurons. However, in the presence of NMDA receptor hypofunction in cortical brainstem projections in patients with schizophrenia, hyperactivity of the mesolimbic dopamine pathway would take place, resulting in excess dopamine and the production of positive symptoms. In addition, under normal conditions, NMDA receptor regulation of mesocortical dopamine pathways is that of tonic excitation. With NMDA receptor hypofunction, the direct result would be hypoactivity of mesocortical dopamine pathways with insufficient dopamine release in the prefrontal cortex, resulting in the cognitive, negative, and affective symptoms of schizophrenia.

In addition to glutamate, glycine is also needed for the NMDA receptor to function. Thus, NMDA receptor functioning can be enhanced by making more glycine available at the synapse, either exogenously by providing glycine or agents that can bind at the glycine site at the NMDA receptor, such as D-serine, D-alanine, and D-cycloserine, or by increasing the availability of endogenous glycine at the synapse through inhibition of the glycine reuptake pump with agents such as sarcosine. All of these strategies have been tested in controlled clinical trials with promising results as evidenced in individual randomized controlled trials [1] and in a meta-analysis of 26 studies [92], except when administered with clozapine, itself a potential glycine transport pump inhibitor [93].

In Phase III of clinical development is bitopertin, a glycine transport inhibitor at the GlyT1 pump site; preliminary results are available for an 8-week, double-blind, placebo-controlled trial [94]. In this trial, clinically stable patients with schizophrenia with predominantly negative symptoms and low severity of positive symptoms were randomized to 10, 30, or 60 mg/day of bitopertin added to ongoing antipsychotic medication treatment. Efficacy (measured by negative symptom severity, overall symptom severity and function) and safety results were considered promising. Studies of bitopertin are ongoing in the following areas/populations: patients with suboptimally controlled symptoms of schizophrenia; persistent, predominant negative symptoms of schizophrenia; biomarker measures of cognitive dysfunction in patients with schizophrenia; and patients with an acute exacerbation of schizophrenia. In most of these trials bitopertin is administered adjunctively with antipsychotics.

Metabotropic glutamate receptors have also been identified as a potential therapeutic target for schizophrenia and a metabotropic glutamate receptor agonist, pomaglumetad methionil, reached Phase III of clinical development [95]. Unfortunately, although the initial randomized controlled clinical trial was positive for monotherapy with this agent

[96], subsequent studies have not been supportive [97,98] and further development has been halted by the manufacturer [99].

Summary

Clozapine remains the standard medication of choice for treatment-resistant schizophrenia. Improvement upon clozapine monotherapy has not been fully demonstrated in clinical trials, although for selected patients the combination of clozapine with other antipsychotics may provide a small additional benefit.

Despite the plethora of randomized controlled trials of putative augmenting agents for treatment-resistant schizophrenia, no single adjunctive agent has been consistently successful in proving efficacy in reducing symptoms, improving cognition, or increasing a patient's level of function. The most promising agents may be antidepressants for negative symptoms. In general, signals for efficacy from small trials have not always been confirmed in larger trials that enroll perhaps more heterogeneous patient samples. Identifying target symptoms may allow for a rational and pragmatic choice among all the adjunctive strategies presented in this review (eg, an antidepressant where negative or depressive symptoms are present), and thus the clinician may want to systematically conduct an "N of 1" trial for a specific individual, being mindful of tolerability and safety issues, in the hopes of achieving a successful outcome.

Few adjunctive agents for schizophrenia have reached Phase III of clinical development; however, drugs that impact glutamate receptors have been the exception. At present there is one candidate remaining in Phase III, a glycine transport inhibitor. If it is successful, it could lead the way for further developments in the field.

References

1 Citrome L. Treatment-refractory schizophrenia: what is it and what has been done about it? *Neuropsychiatry*. 2011;1:325-347.

2 Volavka J, Citrome L. Oral antipsychotics for the treatment of schizophrenia: heterogeneity in efficacy and tolerability should drive decision-making. *Expert Opin Pharmacother*. 2009;10:1917-1928.

3 Novick D, Haro JM, Bertsch J, Haddad PM. Incidence of extrapyramidal symptoms and tardive dyskinesia in schizophrenia: thirty-six-month results from the European schizophrenia outpatient health outcomes study. *J Clin Psychopharmacol*. 2010;30:531-540.

4 Vinogradov S, Fisher M, Warm H, Holland C, Kirshner MA, Pollock BG. The cognitive cost of anticholinergic burden: decreased response to cognitive training in schizophrenia. *Am J Psychiatry*. 2009;166:1055-1062.

5 Leucht S, Corves C, Arbter D, Engel RR, Li C, Davis JM. Second-generation versus first-generation antipsychotic drugs for schizophrenia: a meta-analysis. *Lancet*. 2009;373:31-41.

6 Leucht S, Komossa K, Rummel-Kluge C, et al. A meta-analysis of head-to-head comparisons of second-generation antipsychotics in the treatment of schizophrenia. *Am J Psychiatry*. 2009;166:152-163.

7 Leucht S, Arbter D, Engel RR, Kissling W, Davis JM. How effective are second-generation antipsychotic drugs? A meta-analysis of placebo-controlled trials. *Mol Psychiatry*. 2009;14:429-447.

8 Citrome L. Iloperidone, asenapine, and lurasidone: a brief overview of 3 new second-generation antipsychotics. *Postgrad Med*. 2011;123:153-162.

9 McEvoy JP, Lieberman JA, Stroup TS, et al. Effectiveness of clozapine versus olanzapine, quetiapine, and risperidone in patients with chronic schizophrenia who did not respond to prior atypical antipsychotic treatment. *Am J Psychiatry*. 2006;163:600-610.

10 Volavka J, Czobor P, Sheitman B, et al. Clozapine, olanzapine, risperidone, and haloperidol in the treatment of patients with chronic schizophrenia and schizoaffective disorder. *Am J Psychiatry*. 2002;159:255-262.

11 Kane J, Honigfeld G, Singer J, Meltzer H. Clozapine for the treatment-resistant schizophrenic. A double-blind comparison with chlorpromazine. *Arch Gen Psychiatry*. 1988;45:789-796.

12 Pickar D, Owen RR, Litman RE, Konicki E, Gutierrez R, Rapaport MH. Clinical and biologic response to clozapine in patients with schizophrenia. Crossover comparison with fluphenazine. *Arch Gen Psychiatry*. 1992;49:345-353.

13 Breier A, Buchanan RW, Kirkpatrick B, et al. Effects of clozapine on positive and negative symptoms in outpatients with schizophrenia. *Am J Psychiatry*. 1994;151:20-26.

14 Kumra S, Frazier JA, Jacobsen LK, et al. Childhood-onset schizophrenia. A double-blind clozapine-haloperidol comparison. *Arch Gen Psychiatry*. 1996;53:1090-1097.

15 Hong CJ, Chen JY, Chiu HJ, Sim CB. A double-blind comparative study of clozapine versus chlorpromazine on Chinese patients with treatment-refractory schizophrenia. *Int Clin Psychopharmacol*. 1997;12:123-130.

16 Rosenheck R, Cramer J, Xu W, et al. A comparison of clozapine and haloperidol in hospitalized patients with refractory schizophrenia. Department of Veterans Affairs Cooperative Study Group on Clozapine in Refractory Schizophrenia. *N Engl J Med*. 1997;337:809-815.

17 Buchanan RW, Breier A, Kirkpatrick B, Ball P, Carpenter WT Jr. Positive and negative symptom response to clozapine in schizophrenic patients with and without the deficit syndrome. *Am J Psychiatry*. 1998;155:751-760.

18 Kane JM, Marder SR, Schooler NR, et al. Clozapine and haloperidol in moderately refractory schizophrenia: a 6-month randomized and double-blind comparison. *Arch Gen Psychiatry*. 2001;58:965-972.

19 Bondolfi G, Dufour H, Patris M, et al. Risperidone versus clozapine in treatment-resistant chronic schizophrenia: a randomized double-blind study. The Risperidone Study Group. *Am J Psychiatry*. 1998;155:499-504.

20 Wirshing DA, Marshall BD Jr, Green MF, Mintz J, Marder SR, Wirshing WC. Risperidone in treatment-refractory schizophrenia. *Am J Psychiatry*. 1999;156:1374-1379.

21 Breier AF, Malhotra AK, Su TP, et al. Clozapine and risperidone in chronic schizophrenia: effects on symptoms, parkinsonian side effects, and neuroendocrine response. *Am J Psychiatry*. 1999;156:294-298.

22 Wahlbeck K, Cheine M, Tuisku K, Ahokas A, Joffe G, Rimón R. Risperidone versus clozapine in treatment-resistant schizophrenia: a randomized pilot study. *Prog Neuropsychopharmacol Biol Psychiatry*. 2000;24:911-922.

23 Azorin JM, Spiegel R, Remington G, et al. A double-blind comparative study of clozapine and risperidone in the management of severe chronic schizophrenia. *Am J Psychiatry.* 2001;158:1305-1313.

24 Zhang XY, Zhou DF, Cao LY, Zhang PY, Wu GY, Shen YC. Risperidone versus haloperidol in the treatment of acute exacerbations of chronic inpatients with schizophrenia: a randomized double-blind study. *Int Clin Psychopharmacol.* 2001;16:325-330.

25 Liberman RP, Gutkind D, Mintz J, et al. Impact of risperidone versus haloperidol on activities of daily living in the treatment of refractory schizophrenia. *Compr Psychiatry.* 2002;43:469-473.

26 Conley RR, Kelly DL, Nelson MW, et al. Risperidone, quetiapine, and fluphenazine in the treatment of patients with therapy-refractory schizophrenia. *Clin Neuropharmacol.* 2005;28:163-168.

27 Conley RR, Tamminga CA, Bartko JJ, et al. Olanzapine compared with chlorpromazine in treatment-resistant schizophrenia. *Am J Psychiatry.* 1998;155:914-920.

28 Breier A, Hamilton SH. Comparative efficacy of olanzapine and haloperidol for patients with treatment-resistant schizophrenia. *Biol Psychiatry.* 1999;45:403-411.

29 Tollefson GD, Birkett MA, Kiesler GM, Wood AJ; Lilly Resistant Schizophrenia Study Group. Double-blind comparison of olanzapine versus clozapine in schizophrenic patients clinically eligible for treatment with clozapine. *Biol Psychiatry.* 2001;49:52-63.

30 Conley RR, Kelly DL, Richardson CM, Tamminga CA, Carpenter WT Jr. The efficacy of high-dose olanzapine versus clozapine in treatment-resistant schizophrenia: a double-blind crossover study. *J Clin Psychopharmacol.* 2003;23:668-671.

31 Bitter I, Dossenbach MR, Brook S, et al. Olanzapine versus clozapine in treatment-resistant or treatment -intolerant schizophrenia. *Prog Neuropsychopharmacol Biol Psychiatry.* 2004;28:173-180.

32 Buchanan RW, Ball MP, Weiner E, et al. Olanzapine treatment of residual positive and negative symptoms. *Am J Psychiatry.* 2005;162:124-129.

33 Shaw P, Sporn A, Gogtay N, et al. Childhood-onset schizophrenia: a double-blind, randomized clozapine-olanzapine comparison. *Arch Gen Psychiatry.* 2006;63:721-730.

34 Meltzer HY, Bobo WV, Roy A, et al. A randomized, double-blind comparison of clozapine and high-dose olanzapine in treatment-resistant patients with schizophrenia. *J Clin Psychiatry.* 2008;69:274-285.

35 Kumra S, Kranzler H, Gerbino-Rosen G, et al. Clozapine and "high-dose" olanzapine in refractory early-onset schizophrenia: a 12-week randomized and double-blind comparison. *Biol Psychiatry.* 2008;63:524-529.

36 Emsley RA, Raniwalla J, Bailey PJ, Jones AM; PRIZE Study Group. A comparison of the effects of quetiapine ('seroquel') and haloperidol in schizophrenic patients with a history of and a demonstrated, partial response to conventional antipsychotic treatment. *Int Clin Psychopharmacol.* 2000;15:121-131.

37 Kane JM, Khanna S, Rajadhyaksha S, Giller E. Efficacy and tolerability of ziprasidone in patients with treatment-resistant schizophrenia. *Int Clin Psychopharmacol.* 2006;21:21-28.

38 Sacchetti E, Galluzzo A, Valsecchi P, Romeo F, Gorini B, Warrington L; MOZART Study Group. Ziprasidone vs clozapine in schizophrenia patients refractory to multiple antipsychotic treatments: the MOZART study. *Schizophr Res.* 2009;113:112-121.

39 Kane JM, Meltzer HY, Carson WH Jr, McQuade RD, Marcus RN, Sanchez R; Aripiprazole Study Group. Aripiprazole for treatment-resistant schizophrenia: results of a multicenter, randomized, double-blind, comparison study versus perphenazine. *J Clin Psychiatry.* 2007;68:213-223.

40 Meltzer HY, Alphs L, Green AI, et al; International Suicide Prevention Trial Study Group. Clozapine treatment for suicidality in schizophrenia: International Suicide Prevention Trial (InterSePT). *Arch Gen Psychiatry.* 2003;60:82-91.

41 Krakowski MI, Czobor P, Citrome L, Bark N, Cooper TB. Atypical antipsychotic agents in the treatment of violent patients with schizophrenia and schizoaffective disorder. *Arch Gen Psychiatry* 2006;63:622-629.

42 Lieberman JA, Phillips M, Gu H, et al. Atypical and conventional antipsychotic drugs in treatment-naive first-episode schizophrenia: a 52-week randomized trial of clozapine vs chlorpromazine. *Neuropsychopharmacology.* 2003;28:995-1003.

43 Meltzer HY. Clozapine. *Clin Schizophr Relat Psychoses.* 2012;6:134-144.

44 Schulte PF. Risk of clozapine-associated agranulocytosis and mandatory white blood cell monitoring. *Ann Pharmacother.* 2006;40:683-688.

45 Clozaril® (clozapine) [package insert]. East Hanover, NJ; Novartis Pharmaceuticals Corporation; 2011.

46 Citrome L, Volavka J. Optimal dosing of atypical antipsychotics in adults: a review of the current evidence. *Harv Rev Psychiatry.* 2002;10:280-291.

47 Krakowski M, Czobor P, Citrome L. Weight gain, metabolic parameters, and the impact of race in aggressive inpatients randomized to double-blind clozapine, olanzapine or haloperidol. *Schizophr Res.* 2009;110:95-102.

48 Citrome L, Vreeland B. Schizophrenia, obesity, and antipsychotic medications: what can we do? *Postgrad Med.* 2008;120:18-33.

49 Christison GW, Kirch DG, Wyatt RJ. When symptoms persist: choosing among alternative somatic treatments for schizophrenia. *Schizophr Bull.* 1991;17:217-245.

50 Jaffe AB, Levine J. Antipsychotic medication coprescribing in a large state hospital system. *Pharmacoepidemiol Drug Saf.* 2003;12:41-48.

51 Citrome L, Jaffe A, Levine J. Monotherapy versus polypharmacy for hospitalized psychiatric patients. *Am J Psychiatry.* 2005;162:631.

52 Potter WZ, Ko GN, Zhang LD, Yan WW. Clozapine in China: a review and preview of US/PRC collaboration. *Psychopharmacology (Berl).* 1989;99(suppl):S87-S91.

53 Shiloh R, Zemishlany Z, Aizenberg D, et al. Sulpiride augmentation in people with schizophrenia partially responsive to clozapine. A double-blind, placebo-controlled study. *Br J Psychiatry.* 1997;171:569-573.

54 Josiassen RC, Joseph A, Kohegyi E, et al. Clozapine augmented with risperidone in the treatment of schizophrenia: a randomized, double-blind, placebo-controlled trial. *Am J Psychiatry.* 2005;162:130-136.

55 Anil Yağcioğlu AE, Kivircik Akdede BB, Turgut TI, et al. A double-blind controlled study of adjunctive treatment with risperidone in schizophrenic patients partially responsive to clozapine: efficacy and safety. *J Clin Psychiatry.* 2005;66:63-72.

56 Honer WG, Thornton AE, Chen EY, et al; Clozapine and Risperidone Enhancement (CARE) Study Group. Clozapine alone versus clozapine and risperidone with refractory schizophrenia. *N Engl J Med.* 2006;354:472-482.

57 Freudenreich O, Henderson DC, Walsh JP, Culhane MA, Goff DC. Risperidone augmentation for schizophrenia partially responsive to clozapine: a double-blind, placebo-controlled trial. *Schizophr Res.* 2007;92:90-94.

58 Weiner E, Conley RR, Ball MP, et al. Adjunctive risperidone for partially responsive people with schizophrenia treated with clozapine. *Neuropsychopharmacology.* 2010;35:2274-2283.

59 Kreinin A, Novitski D, Weizman A. Amisulpride treatment of clozapine-induced hypersalivation in schizophrenia patients: a randomized, double-blind, placebo-controlled cross-over study. *Int Clin Psychopharmacol.* 2006;21:99-103.

60 Assion HJ, Reinbold H, Lemanski S, Basilowski M, Juckel G. Amisulpride augmentation in patients with schizophrenia partially responsive or unresponsive to clozapine. A randomized, double-blind, placebo-controlled trial. *Pharmacopsychiatry.* 2008;41:24-28.

61 Genç Y, Taner E, Candansayar S. Comparison of clozapine-amisulpride and clozapine-quetiapine combinations for patients with schizophrenia who are partially responsive to clozapine: a single-blind randomized study. *Adv Ther.* 2007;24:1-13.

62 Chang JS, Ahn YM, Park HJ, et al. Aripiprazole augmentation in clozapine-treated patients with refractory schizophrenia: an 8-week, randomized, double-blind, placebo-controlled trial. *J Clin Psychiatry.* 2008;69:720-731.

63 Fleischhacker WW, Heikkinen ME, Olié JP, et al. Effects of adjunctive treatment with aripiprazole on body weight and clinical efficacy in schizophrenia patients treated with clozapine: a randomized, double-blind, placebo-controlled trial. *Int J Neuropsychopharmacol.* 2010;13:1115-1125.

64 Muscatello MR, Bruno A, Pandolfo G, et al. Effect of aripiprazole augmentation of clozapine in schizophrenia: a double-blind, placebo-controlled study. *Schizophr Res.* 2011;127:93-99.

65 Zink M, Kuwilsky A, Krumm B, Dressing H. Efficacy and tolerability of ziprasidone versus risperidone as augmentation in patients partially responsive to clozapine: a randomised controlled clinical trial. *J Psychopharmacol.* 2009;23:305-314.

66 Kane JM, Correll CU, Goff DC, et al. A multicenter, randomized, double-blind, placebo-controlled, 16-week study of adjunctive aripiprazole for schizophrenia or schizoaffective disorder inadequately treated with quetiapine or risperidone monotherapy. *J Clin Psychiatry.* 2009;70:1348-1357.

67 Henderson DC, Fan X, Copeland PM, et al. Aripiprazole added to overweight and obese olanzapine-treated schizophrenia patients. *J Clin Psychopharmacol.* 2009;29:165-169.

68 Shafti SS. Augmentation of olanzapine by fluphenazine decanoate in poorly responsive schizophrenia. *Clin Schizophr Relat Psychoses.* 2009;3:97-102.

69 Kotler M, Strous RD, Reznik I, Shwartz S, Weizman A, Spivak B. Sulpiride augmentation of olanzapine in the management of treatment-resistant chronic schizophrenia: evidence for improvement of mood symptomatology. *Int Clin Psychopharmacol.* 2004;19:23-26.

70 Takahashi N, Terao T, Oga T, Okada M. Comparison of risperidone and mosapramine addition to neuroleptic treatment in chronic schizophrenia. *Neuropsychobiology.* 1999;39:81-85.

71 Cipriani A, Boso M, Barbui C. Clozapine combined with different antipsychotic drugs for treatment resistant schizophrenia. *Cochrane Database Syst Rev.* 2009;(3):CD006324.

72 Taylor DM, Smith L, Gee SH, Nielsen J. Augmentation of clozapine with a second antipsychotic – a meta-analysis. *Acta Psychiatr Scand.* 2012;125:15-24.

73 Citrome L, Levine J, Allingham B. Changes in use of valproate and other mood stabilizers for patients with schizophrenia from 1994 to 1998. *Psychiatr Serv.* 2000;51:634-638.

74 Citrome L, Jaffe A, Levine J, Allingham B. Use of mood stabilizers among patients with schizophrenia, 1994-2001. *Psychiatr Serv.* 2002;53:1212.

75 Citrome L. Use of lithium, carbamazepine, and valproic acid in a state-operated psychiatric hospital. *J Pharm Technol.* 1995;11:55-59.

76 Citrome L. Adjunctive lithium and anticonvulsants for the treatment of schizophrenia: what is the evidence? *Expert Rev Neurother.* 2009;9:55-71.

77 Tiihonen J, Wahlbeck K, Kiviniemi V. The efficacy of lamotrigine in clozapine-resistant schizophrenia: a systematic review and meta-analysis. *Schizophr Res.* 2009;109:10-14.

78 Citrome L, Shope CB, Nolan KA, Czobor P, Volavka J. Risperidone alone versus risperidone plus valproate in the treatment of patients with schizophrenia and hostility. *Int Clin Psychopharmacol.* 2007;22:356-362.

79 Volavka J, Citrome L. Heterogeneity of violence in schizophrenia and implications for long-term treatment. *Int J Clin Pract.* 2008;62:1237-1245.

80 Volavka J, Citrome L. Pathways to aggression in schizophrenia affect results of treatment. *Schizophr Bull.* 2011;37:921-929.

81 Citrome L, Volavka J. Pharmacological management of acute and persistent aggression in forensic psychiatry settings. *CNS Drugs.* 2011;25:1009-1021.

82 Buckley P, Citrome L, Nichita C, Vitacco M. Psychopharmacology of aggression in schizophrenia. *Schizophr Bull.* 2011;37:930-936.

83 Nolan KA, Citrome L. Reducing inpatient aggression: does paying attention pay off? *Psychiatr Q.* 2008;79:91-95.

84 Grohmann R, Engel RR, Geissler KH, Rüther E. Psychotropic drug use in psychiatric inpatients: recent trends and changes over time-data from the AMSP study. *Pharmacopsychiatry.* 2004;37(suppl 1):S27-S28.

85 Xiang Y-T, Ungvari GS, Wang C-Y, et al. Adjunctive antidepressant prescriptions for hospitalized patients with schizophrenia in Asia (2001–2009). *Asia Pac Psychiatry*. Epub 29 Aug 2012.

86 Conley RR. The burden of depressive symptoms in people with schizophrenia. *Psychiatr Clin North Am*. 2009;32:853-861.

87 Makinen J, Miettunen J, Isohanni M, Koponen H. Negative symptoms in schizophrenia: a review. *Nord J Psychiatry*. 2008;62:334-341.

88 Singh SP, Singh V, Kar N, Chan K. Efficacy of antidepressants in treating the negative symptoms of chronic schizophrenia: meta-analysis. *Br J Psychiatry*. 2010;197:174-179.

89 Lieberman JA, Dunbar G, Segreti AC, et al. A randomized exploratory trial of an alpha-7 nicotinic receptor agonist (TC-5619) for cognitive enhancement in schizophrenia. *Neuropsychopharmacology*. 2013. In press.

90 Freedman R, Olincy A, Buchanan RW, et al. Initial phase 2 trial of a nicotinic agonist in schizophrenia. *Am J Psychiatry* 2008;165:1040-1047.

91 Kantrowitz J, Javitt DC. Glutamatergic transmission in schizophrenia: from basic research to clinical practice. *Curr Opin Psychiatry*. 2012;25:96-102.

92 Tsai GE, Lin PY. Strategies to enhance N-methyl-D-aspartate receptor-mediated neurotransmission in schizophrenia, a critical review and meta-analysis. *Curr Pharm Des*. 2010;16:522-537.

93 Javitt DC, Duncan L, Balla A, Sershen H. Inhibition of System A-mediated glycine transport in cortical synaptosomes by therapeutic concentrations of clozapine: implications for mechanisms of action. *Mol Psychiatry*. 2005;10:275-287.

94 Umbricht D, Yoo K, Youssef E, et al. Investigational glycine transporter type 1 (GlyT1) inhibitor RG1678: results of the proof-of-concept study for the treatment of negative symptoms in schizophrenia. Poster presented at: 49th Annual Meeting of the American College of Neuropsychopharmacology; December 5–9, 2010; Miami Beach, FL.

95 Kinon BJ, Gómez JC. Clinical development of pomaglumetad methionil: A non-dopaminergic treatment for schizophrenia. *Neuropharmacology*. 2013;66:82-86.

96 Patil ST, Zhang L, Martenyi F, et al. Activation of mGlu2/3 receptors as a new approach to treat schizophrenia: a randomized Phase 2 clinical trial. *Nat Med*. 2007;13:1102-1107.

97 Kinon BJ, Zhang L, Millen BA, et al; and the HBBI Study Group. A multicenter, inpatient, phase 2, double-blind, placebo-controlled dose-ranging study of LY2140023 monohydrate in patients with DSM-IV schizophrenia. *J Clin Psychopharmacol*. 2011;31:349-355.

98 Lilly announces pomaglumetad methionil did not meet primary endpoint of clinical study [press release]. Eli Lilly and Company; July 11, 2012. newsroom.lilly.com/releasedetail.cfm?ReleaseID=690836. Accessed March 19, 2013.

99 Lilly stops Phase III development of pomaglumetad methionil for the treatment of schizophrenia based on efficacy results [press release]. Eli Lilly and Company; August 29, 2012. newsroom.lilly.com/releasedetail.cfm?ReleaseID=703018. Accessed March 19, 2013.

Chapter 6

Somatic treatments

Nonpharmacologic interventions that are used in combination with antipsychotic medications include somatic therapies such as electroconvulsive therapy (ECT), repetitive transcranial magnetic stimulation (rTMS), and acupuncture. Table 6.1 lists several randomized controlled trials of ECT and rTMS in patients with persistent symptoms of schizophrenia [1–14].

Adjunctive ECT has been tested in randomized controlled trials [2,3], and its use with clozapine is encouraging [15]. However, the bulk of supporting evidence for ECT in treatment-resistant schizophrenia is found in uncontrolled studies [16–21].

More than ten randomized controlled trials of rTMS in patients with persistent symptoms of schizophrenia have been published, but the results of the individual studies are mixed [4–14]. In a meta-analysis of nine trials [22], the effect size for treating negative symptoms of schizophrenia for prefrontal rTMS versus sham was statistically significant and in the small-to-medium range. When including only the studies using a frequency of stimulation of 10 Hz, the effect size increased; when including only the studies requiring participants to be on a stable drug regimen before and during the study, the effect size decreased. Studies with a longer duration of treatment (≥ 3 weeks) had a larger effect size when compared to studies with shorter treatment duration [22]. Another meta-analysis of prospective studies of rTMS in refractory schizophrenia assessed the effects of high-frequency rTMS to the left dorsolateral prefrontal cortex for the treatment of negative symptoms and low-frequency rTMS to the left

L. Citrome, *Handbook of Treatment-resistant Schizophrenia*,
DOI: 10.1007/978-1-908517-88-3_6,
© Springer Healthcare 2013

temporoparietal cortex for the treatment of auditory hallucinations and overall positive symptoms; the sham-controlled studies did not support the use of rTMS for negative or positive symptoms (the small effect size was not statistically significant) [23]. However, when specifically examining

Antipsychotic medication plus somatic nonpharmacological interventions in patients with schizophrenia				
Author and year	**Study duration**	**Number randomized**	**Intervention**	**Comments***
Chanpattana 1999 [2]	6 months	51	ECT and flupenthixol	ECT and flupenthixol > ECT or flupenthixol
Goswami 2003 [3]	4 weeks	25	ECT and chlorpromazine	ECT and chlorpromazine > chlorpromazine
McIntosh 2004 [4]	4 days	16	rTMS and one or more antipsychotics	rTMS and one or more antipsychotics ~ one or more antipsychotics
Fitzgerald 2005 [5]	10 weeks	33	rTMS and second-generation antipsychotic	rTMS and second-generation antipsychotic ~ second-generation antipsychotic
Lee 2005 [6]	10 days	39	rTMS and antipsychotic	rTMS and antipsychotic > antipsychotic
Saba 2006 [7]	10 days	18	rTMS and antipsychotic	rTMS and antipsychotic ~ antipsychotic
Mogg 2007 [8]	10 days	17	rTMS and antipsychotic	rTMS and antipsychotic ~ antipsychotic
Prikryl 2007 [9]	15 days	22	rTMS and antipsychotic	rTMS and antipsychotic > antipsychotic
Rosa 2007 [10]	10 days	11	rTMS and clozapine	rTMS and clozapine ~ clozapine
Fitzgerald 2008 [11]	3 weeks	29	rTMS and antipsychotic	rTMS and antipsychotic ~ antipsychotic
Schneider 2008 [12]	4 weeks	51	rTMS and second-generation antipsychotic	rTMS and second-generation antipsychotic > second-generation antipsychotic
Vercammen 2009 [13]	6 days	38	rTMS and antipsychotic	rTMS and antipsychotic > antipsychotic
De Jesus 2010 [14]	20 days	17	rTMS and clozapine	rTMS and clozapine > clozapine

Table 6.1 Antipsychotic medication plus somatic nonpharmacological interventions in patients with schizophrenia. As tested in randomized controlled trials with an emphasis on persistent symptoms despite antipsychotic treatment. *In some studies, multiple different outcomes were measured and some small differences may have emerged that are different from the overall results as noted here. ~, means similar to or no difference from. ECT, electroconvulsive therapy; rTMS, repetitive transcranial magnetic stimulation. Reproduced with permission from Citrome [1].

auditory hallucinations, the effect size for the sham-controlled studies was large and statistically significant [23].

Acupuncture is another physical modality that has been tested in patients with schizophrenia. A systematic review evaluated 13 randomized controlled trials of acupuncture for schizophrenia, all originating from China [24]; the authors noted that methodological quality was generally poor and that firm conclusions could not be made. One of the 13 studies reported significant effects of electroacupuncture plus drug therapy for improving auditory hallucinations and positive symptoms compared with sham electroacupuncture plus drug therapy. Seven studies showed significant effects of acupuncture plus antipsychotic drug therapy for response compared with antipsychotic drug therapy alone. Two studies tested laser acupuncture against sham laser acupuncture with one finding beneficial effects of laser acupuncture on hallucinations and the other study showing significant effects of laser acupuncture on response rate, Brief Psychiatric Rating Scale, and clinical global index compared with sham laser.

Summary

Among the nonpharmacological modalities described in this chapter, ECT is the oldest and most well-known. The evidence supporting the use of ECT in the management of patients with treatment-resistant schizophrenia is largely limited to uncontrolled studies and case reports. Logistical and technical challenges in designing and implementing randomized controlled trials of adjunctive ECT probably explain why they are rare. Nevertheless, where available, ECT should at least be considered. rTMS is somewhat easier to study; results so far, however, are not compelling enough to recommend its routine use in treatment-resistant schizophrenia.

References

1   Citrome L. Treatment-refractory schizophrenia: what is it and what has been done about it? *Neuropsychiatry*. 2011;1:325-347.

2   Chanpattana W, Chakrabhand ML, Sackeim HA, et al. Continuation ECT in treatment-resistant schizophrenia: a controlled study. *J ECT*. 1999;15:178-192.

3   Goswami U, Kumar U, Singh B. Efficacy of electroconvulsive therapy in treatment resistant schizophrenia: a double blind study. *Indian J Psychiatry*. 2003;45:26-29.

4   McIntosh AM, Semple D, Tasker K, et al. Transcranial magnetic stimulation for auditory hallucinations in schizophrenia. *Psychiatry Res*. 2004;127:9-17.

5   Fitzgerald PB, Benitez J, Daskalakis JZ, et al. A double-blind sham-controlled trial of repetitive transcranial magnetic stimulation in the treatment of refractory auditory hallucinations. *J Clin Psychopharmacol*. 2005;25:358-362.

6   Lee SH, Kim W, Chung YC, et al. A double blind study showing that two weeks of daily repetitive TMS over the left or right temporoparietal cortex reduces symptoms in patients with schizophrenia who are having treatment-refractory auditory hallucinations. *Neurosci Lett*. 2005;376:177-181.

7   Saba G, Verdon CM, Kalalou K, et al. Transcranial magnetic stimulation in the treatment of schizophrenic symptoms: a double blind sham controlled study. *J Psychiatr Res*. 2006;40:147-152.

8   Mogg A, Purvis R, Eranti S, et al. Repetitive transcranial magnetic stimulation for negative symptoms of schizophrenia: a randomized controlled pilot study. *Schizophr Res*. 2007;93:221-228.

9   Prikryl R, Kasparek T, Skotakova S, Ustohal L, Kucerova H, Ceskova E. Treatment of negative symptoms of schizophrenia using repetitive transcranial magnetic stimulation in a double-blind, randomized controlled study. *Schizophr Res*. 2007;95:151-157.

10 Rosa MO, Gattaz WF, Rosa MA, et al. Effects of repetitive transcranial magnetic stimulation on auditory hallucinations refractory to clozapine. *J Clin Psychiatry*. 2007;68:1528-1532.

11 Fitzgerald PB, Herring S, Hoy K, et al. A study of the effectiveness of bilateral transcranial magnetic stimulation in the treatment of the negative symptoms of schizophrenia. *Brain Stimul*. 2008;1:27-32.

12 Schneider AL, Schneider TL, Stark H. Repetitive transcranial magnetic stimulation (rTMS) as an augmentation treatment for the negative symptoms of schizophrenia: A 4-week randomized placebo controlled study. *Brain Stimul*. 2008;1:106-111.

13 Vercammen A, Knegtering H, Bruggeman R, et al. Effects of bilateral repetitive transcranial magnetic stimulation on treatment resistant auditory-verbal hallucinations in schizophrenia: a randomized controlled trial. *Schizophr Res*. 2009;114:172-179.

14 de Jesus DR, Gil A, Barbosa L, et al. A pilot double-blind sham-controlled trial of repetitive transcranial magnetic stimulation for patients with refractory schizophrenia treated with clozapine. *Psychiatry Res*. 2011;188:203-207.

15 Braga RJ, Petrides G. The combined use of electroconvulsive therapy and antipsychotics in patients with schizophrenia. *J ECT*. 2005;21:75-83.

16 Garg R, Chavan BS, Arun P. Quality of life after electroconvulsive therapy in persons with treatment resistant schizophrenia. *Indian J Med Res* 2011;133:641-644.

17 Ravanic DB, Pantovic MM, Milovanovic DR, et al. Long-term efficacy of electroconvulsive therapy combined with different antipsychotic drugs in previously resistant schizophrenia. *Psychiatr Danub*. 2009;21:179-186.

18 Kho KH, Blansjaar BA, de Vries S, Babuskova D, Zwinderman AH, Linszen DH. Electroconvulsive therapy for the treatment of clozapine nonresponders suffering from schizophrenia – an open label study. *Eur Arch Psychiatry Clin Neurosci*. 2004;254:372-379.

19 Levy-Rueff M, Gourevitch R, Loo H, Olie JP, Amado I. Maintenance electroconvulsive therapy: an alternative treatment for refractory schizophrenia and schizoaffective disorders. *Psychiatry Res*. 2010;175:280-283.

20 Tang WK, Ungvari G. Efficacy of electroconvulsive therapy combined with antipsychotic medication in treatment-resistant schizophrenia: a prospective, open trial. *J ECT*. 2002;18:90-94.

21 Chanpattana W, Andrade C. ECT for treatment-resistant schizophrenia: a response from the far East to the UK. NICE report. *J ECT*. 2006;22:4-12.

22 Dlabac-de Lange JJ, Knegtering R, Aleman A. Repetitive transcranial magnetic stimulation for negative symptoms of schizophrenia: review and meta-analysis. *J Clin Psychiatry*. 2010;71:411-418.

23 Freitas C, Fregni F, Pascual-Leone A. Meta-analysis of the effects of repetitive transcranial magnetic stimulation (rTMS) on negative and positive symptoms in schizophrenia. *Schizophr Res*. 2009;108:11-24.

24 Lee MS, Shin BC, Ronan P, Ernst E. Acupuncture for schizophrenia: a systematic review and meta-analysis. *Int J Clin Pract*. 2009;63:1622-1633.

Chapter 7

Nonpharmacological approaches

Cognitive behavioral therapy and cognitive remediation

Cognitive-behavioral therapy (CBT), although labor-intensive, can be helpful even in patients considered treatment-refractory, and has been evaluated in controlled clinical trials in patients with treatment-resistant schizophrenia [1–3]. In a 6-month randomized controlled trial comparing CBT plus social skills training and clozapine versus supportive therapy and clozapine in 41 patients, subjects who had received CBT plus social skills training had lower psychopathology scores than those who received supportive therapy [1]. In a 21-week controlled but nonrandomized trial with 21 patients comparing CBT plus clozapine versus befriending plus clozapine, the CBT group showed a significant improvement in psychopathology and quality of life, and the improvement in psychopathology persisted at the 6-month follow-up assessment [2]. However, mixed results were found in another controlled study comparing CBT versus counseling in 62 patients taking at least one atypical antipsychotic (mostly clozapine) [3]. Patients receiving CBT had improved with regard to auditory hallucinations and illness insight at the post-treatment assessment, but these findings were not maintained at follow-up.

Cognitive remediation is a set of drills or compensatory interventions designed to enhance cognitive functioning; it is a therapy which engages the patient in learning activities that enhance the neurocognitive skills relevant to their chosen recovery goals [4]. Moderate range effect sizes

L. Citrome, *Handbook of Treatment-resistant Schizophrenia*,
DOI: 10.1007/978-1-908517-88-3_7,
© Springer Healthcare 2013

on cognitive test performance and daily functioning have been reported in six meta-analyses [4,5]. There is heterogeneity in patient response to cognitive remediation and this is dependent on baseline abilities, motivation, and the techniques used. The behavioral treatments specifically target memory, attention, executive functioning, and reasoning. Restorative cognitive techniques include drills, practices with paper and pencil tasks, and computerized training software, used individually and in groups. The promotion of adaptive behavior by compensatory cognitive training is believed to help enhance daily functioning at school, work, in social interactions, and in independent living [4]. In a randomized controlled study of cognitive remediation among 85 inpatients at a state-operated psychiatric hospital, patients in the cognitive remediation group demonstrated significantly greater improvements over 3 months than the control group in the composite measure of overall cognitive functioning, psychomotor speed, and verbal learning; notably, patients in both groups showed significant and comparable improvements over the follow-up period on the positive, activation, and depression factors of the Positive and Negative Syndrome Scale [6].

Psychosocial rehabilitation, vocational rehabilitation, and supported employment

Components of psychosocial rehabilitation include the improvement of neurocognition (attention, processing, memory, reasoning, verbal learning, visual learning), social cognition (emotion processing, social perception, attributional bias, theory of mind), motivation (external, intrinsic), and ultimately functional and subjective outcomes [7]. Although CBT techniques and cognitive remediation are integral to psychosocial rehabilitation, a key issue that needs to be addressed is patient employment. Although most people with schizophrenia are unemployed, most do identify employment as a goal [7].

Barriers to employment include cognitive impairments, psychiatric symptoms, substance use, nonpsychiatric medical conditions, stigma from employers, internalized stigma and low self-confidence, and the fear of losing disability benefits [7,8]. Vocational rehabilitation addresses these barriers by providing skill training, sheltered workshops, transitional employment, and supported employment [7,8]. Basic principles of supported employment are zero exclusion with eligibility based on consumer choice, focus on competitive jobs in integrated community settings, rapid job searches, respect for consumers' preferences in terms of the nature of the job and types of support services, ongoing job support, close integration with a psychosocial rehabilitation team approach, and benefits counseling (disability benefits, Social Security, medical insurance) [8].

In a randomized controlled trial evaluating the effects of adding cognitive remediation to a vocational rehabilitation program compared with vocational rehabilitation alone in 34 people with severe mental illness, patients who received both cognitive remediation and vocational rehabilitation demonstrated significantly greater improvements on a cognitive battery over 3 months than those who received vocational rehabilitation alone, and had better work outcomes over the 2-year follow-up period [8]. With employment one may expect increased self-esteem, reduction in symptoms and hospitalizations, enhanced social functioning, and improvement in overall quality of life [7,8].

Other approaches

Other psychological and behavioral interventions that have been tested in randomized controlled trials and have demonstrated potential utility in treatment-refractory schizophrenia include hallucination-focused integrative treatment [9], targeted cognitive training [10], and occupational therapy [11]. In an 18-month study, 63 patients received hallucination-focused integrative treatment and an antipsychotic versus an antipsychotic alone [9]. Subjects in the experimental group retained improvements over time. Improvements in hallucinations, distress, and negative content of voices remained significant. In a 6-month study (N = 32) of targeted cognitive training combined with medication versus a computer games control condition combined with medication, subjects receiving targeted cognitive training showed significant durable gains [10]. In a 6-month study (N = 26) comparing occupational therapy plus clozapine versus clozapine alone found that the occupational therapy intervention was effective in terms of occupational performance and interpersonal relationships mainly from the fourth month to the end of the study [11].

Summary

CBT and cognitive remediation, when available, can improve a person's opportunity for being in recovery. The combination of cognitive remediation and vocational rehabilitation provides superior outcomes compared with vocational rehabilitation alone.

References

1 Pinto A, La Pia S, Mennella R, Giorgio D, DeSimone L. Cognitive-behavioral therapy and clozapine for clients with treatment-refractory schizophrenia. *Psychiatr Serv*. 1999;50:901-904.
2 Barretto EM, Kayo M, Avrichir BS, et al. A preliminary controlled trial of cognitive behavioral therapy in clozapine-resistant schizophrenia. *J Nerv Ment Dis*. 2009;197:865-868.
3 Valmaggia LR, van der Gaag M, Tarrier N, Pijnenborg M, Slooff CJ. Cognitive-behavioural therapy for refractory psychotic symptoms of schizophrenia resistant to atypical antipsychotic medication. Randomised controlled trial. *Br J Psychiatry*. 2005;186:324-330.
4 Medalia A, Choi J. Cognitive remediation in schizophrenia. *Neuropsychol Rev*. 2009;19:353-364.
5 Kurtz MM. Cognitive remediation for schizophrenia: current status, biological correlates and predictors of response. *Expert Rev Neurother*. 2012;12:813-821.
6 Lindenmayer JP, McGurk SR, Mueser KT, et al. A randomized controlled trial of cognitive remediation among inpatients with persistent mental illness. *Psychiatr Serv*. 2008;59:241-247.
7 Kurzban S, Davis L, Brekke JS. Vocational, social, and cognitive rehabilitation for individuals diagnosed with schizophrenia: a review of recent research and trends. *Curr Psychiatry Rep*. 2010;12:345-355.
8 McGurk SR, Mueser KT, DeRosa TJ, Wolfe R. Work, recovery, and comorbidity in schizophrenia: a randomized controlled trial of cognitive remediation. *Schizophr Bull*. 2009;35:319-335.
9 Jenner JA, Nienhuis FJ, van de Willige G, Wiersma D. "Hitting" voices of schizophrenia patients may lastingly reduce persistent auditory hallucinations and their burden: 18-month outcome of a randomized controlled trial. *Can J Psychiatry*. 2006;51:169-177.
10 Fisher M, Holland C, Subramaniam K, Vinogradov S. Neuroplasticity-based cognitive training in schizophrenia: an interim report on the effects 6 months later. *Schizophr Bull*. 2010;36:869-879.
11 Buchain PC, Vizzotto AD, Henna Neto J, Elkis H. Randomized controlled trial of occupational therapy in patients with treatment-resistant schizophrenia. *Rev Bras Psiquiatr*. 2003;25:26-30.

Chapter 8

Conclusions

It is a fact that not all people with schizophrenia respond equally well to all treatments. In circling back to the principles of evidence-based medicine, we need to recognize the uniqueness of individuals and that "one size does *not* fit all." The first step in assessing treatment response or lack thereof is the comprehensive and accurate identification of barriers to successful treatment. This may include partial or nonadherence, alcohol or substance use, or inadequate antipsychotic doses or inadequate antipsychotic plasma levels. The best tool available is the therapeutic alliance, which can be further enhanced by using the techniques of motivational interviewing.

Schizophrenia is a multidimensional disease with several treatment domains: positive symptoms, negative symptoms, depression/anxiety, excitement/hostility, and cognitive dysfunction. For many patients hallucinations and delusions may not be as functionally disabling as negative symptoms or cognitive dysfunction. Moreover, the symptom domain of depression and anxiety may be of particular interest and concern to the individual patient, and the symptom domain of excitement/hostility has been a frequent reason for hospitalization. Lack of adequate treatment response can be either global or restricted to one of these specific domains. The identification of specific target symptoms must be individualized, and in addition to psychotic symptoms, other symptoms that the patient finds significant are important to make explicit. Other patient-centered concerns are potential tolerability issues that may have interfered with

L. Citrome, *Handbook of Treatment-resistant Schizophrenia*,
DOI: 10.1007/978-1-908517-88-3_8,
© Springer Healthcare 2013

adherence and response in the past. When selecting a potential adjunctive treatment, new tolerability concerns can potentially complicate expectations and outcomes.

Clozapine remains the antipsychotic medication of choice when other antipsychotics have failed. Psychosocial rehabilitation can assist in improving functionality and enhance the opportunity for recovery. Improvement upon clozapine monotherapy remains elusive to demonstrate in clinical trials, although for selected patients the combination of clozapine with other antipsychotics may provide a small additional benefit. Clinical trials of adjunctive/augmentation strategies of antipsychotics with other medications have not yet yielded a new standard of care, but do provide signals that adjunctive antidepressants and possibly adjunctive agents that impact on glutamate receptors may be helpful. Optimistically, having different medication interventions with different potential mechanisms of action may facilitate identifying subtypes of schizophrenia that can guide rational treatment selection.

Printed by Books on Demand, Germany